COMBAT MEDICINE

OPERATIONS MANUAL

COVER IMAGE: **Security force team members for Provincial Reconstruction Team (PRT) Farah wait for a UH-60 Blackhawk MEDEVAC helicopter to land before moving a simulated casualty during medical evacuation training on FOB Farah, Afghanistan, 9 January 2013.**
(US Navy photo/HMC Josh Ives)

Dedication

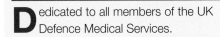

Dedicated to all members of the UK Defence Medical Services.

First published in October 2019

A catalogue record for this book is available from the British Library.

ISBN 978 1 78521 265 9

Library of Congress control no. 2019634678

Published by Haynes Publishing,
Sparkford, Yeovil, Somerset BA22 7JJ, UK.
Tel: 01963 440635
Int. tel: +44 1963 440635
Website: www.haynes.com

Haynes North America Inc.,
859 Lawrence Drive, Newbury Park,
California 91320, USA.

Printed in Malaysia.

Senior Commissioning Editor: Jonathan Falconer
Copy editor: Michelle Tilling
Proof reader: Penny Housden
Indexer: Peter Nicholson
Page design: James Robertson

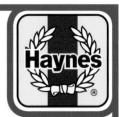

COMBAT MEDICINE

OPERATIONS MANUAL

From the Korean War to Afghanistan

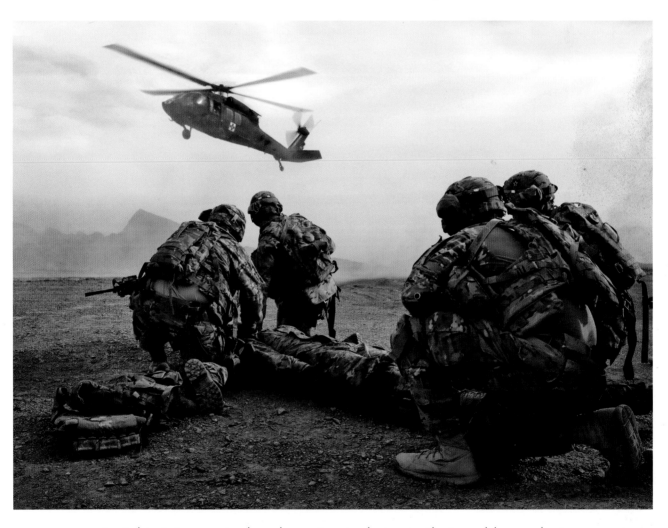

Insights into surgical and nursing techniques that enable combat
medical teams to save lives and alleviate suffering on the battlefield

Penny Starns

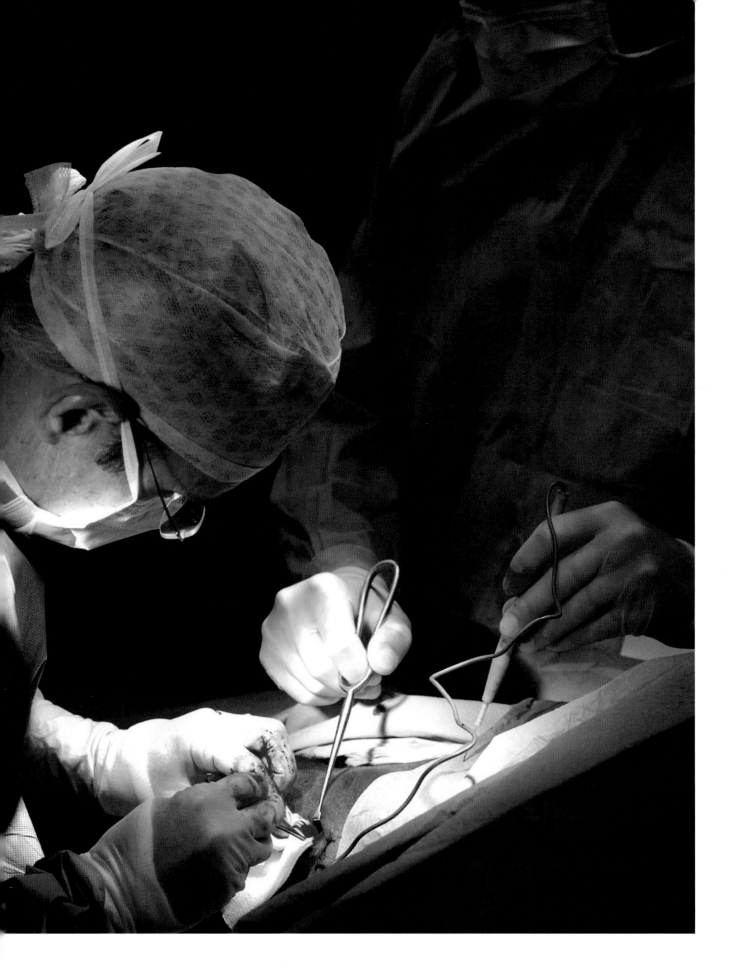

Contents

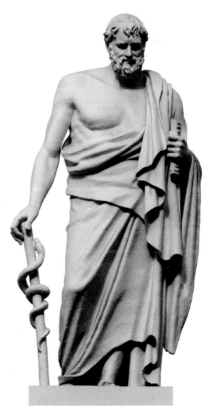

OPPOSITE A surgeon operates on a patient with a gunshot wound at the Camp Bastion Medical Facility in Helmand, Afghanistan, during 2007. *(MOD Open Government Licence)*

RIGHT In Western culture the great ancient Greek physician Hippocrates is often called the father of medicine. The Hippocratic Oath, traditionally sworn by all new physicians, includes the vow to '… use treatment to help the sick according to my ability and judgment, but never with a view to injury and wrong-doing'. *(Shutterstock)*

Acknowledgements

It has been an enormous privilege to write about the life and work of combat medics, and I thank my editor Jonathan Falconer for his enthusiastic interest in the subject matter and unequivocal support. Professor Ronald Hutton and Dr Victoria Bates of the University of Bristol deserve a special mention for providing me with practical assistance and intellectual stimulation, through the dynamic and thought-provoking activities of the Medical Humanities Department. Part-way through the writing process I experienced serious computer problems. Fortunately, these were calmly and efficiently resolved by Raf Iwo Jarzebski, also of the University of Bristol, and I am extremely grateful to him for his expertise in the field of information technology.

The research for this book has been greatly assisted by combat medics past and present. In this respect I am indebted to Captain Jane Titley, ARRC Matron-in-Chief of Queen Alexandra's Royal Naval Nursing Service 1991–94, Colonel Gruber Von Arni ARRC of the Queen Alexandra's Royal Army Nursing Service and the late Dr Monica Baly of the Princess Mary's Royal Air Force Nursing Service for giving me valuable insights into the history and work of military nursing services. In more recent times

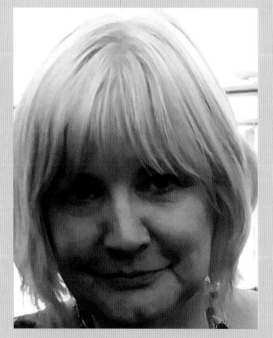

RIGHT Dr Penny Starns, the author.

other military medics have generously contributed their time, thoughts and knowledge to my research. For his wonderful assistance I thank Jay Myers of the RAF Media and Publicity Department. Jay cheerfully and quickly opened numerous official doors, through his extensive communications network, which would otherwise have remained closed.

Special thanks are due to Wing Commander Bob Tipping, Consultant Adviser in Pre-hospital Care to Hd RAFMS, and Lieutenant Colonel Harvey Pynn RAMC, Defence Consultant Advisor in Pre-hospital Emergency Care, for patiently reading some of the chapters and kindly providing me with valuable feedback on the text. I am also appreciative of the further information provided by Wing Commander Andrew Davy, RAF Command Flight Medical Officer RAF Centre of Aviation Medicine, Wing Commander Peter Hodkinson, Consultant in Aviation and Space Medicine and Squadron Leader Garth Logan, SO2 Aeromed, Aeromedical Evacuation Control Centre. Collectively this team ensured that I had access to unique and fascinating primary source material.

When it came to finding photographs and illustrations for this book there are several people who assisted my efforts. For pointing me in the right direction to obtain crucial trauma pathway diagrams I thank Dr Simon Mercer, Consultant Anaesthetist at Aintree University and Defence Lecturer in Anaesthesia at the National Institute of Academic Anaesthesia. Additionally, Richard Hieron of the Ministry of Defence deserves a mention for his persistence in dealing with my permissions requests. Iain Moir of the National Institute for Clinical Excellence gave me timely and pertinent advice, and staff at the Imperial War Museum image library were very helpful. I am also grateful to David Coates of the Air Sector Communications department of BAE Systems, for providing me with images of the latest protective helmets for Typhoon pilots.

Finally, I thank the Haynes editorial, design and production team for assembling the text, photographs and illustrations in their own stylish, inimitable way. They, and the combat medics themselves, are the people who make this a truly remarkable manual.

Introduction

Battlefield medicine – a personal journey in research

The process of research and writing for this manual has been essentially a medical pilgrimage and a labour of love. It provides unique historical insights into the heroic life-saving work of combat medics. In addition to documenting numerous human stories of conflict and the history of battlefield medicine it also contains powerful and profoundly moving archival images.

From the outset I was thankful for the military personnel who had earlier assisted my PhD research and for my own medical background. Furthermore, being a complete newcomer to the art of finding and scrutinising appropriate images to illustrate text, I was grateful to receive pertinent advice from my commissioning editor at Haynes, Jonathan Falconer, who has considerable expertise in this area.

In terms of research approaches, my first thoughts centred on how best to structure the material in a way that would make sense to the reader. Among the detailed instruction tables, facts and figures, it was important to highlight historical developments in combat medical support, first response training, medical specialism, evacuation procedures, anaesthesia and surgical techniques, combat stress and current military research. However, when military medics are dealing with wounded personnel in war zones everything happens instantaneously, and this sense of urgency in combat casualty care needed to be conveyed within the text.

Once the framework was in place I undertook image and text research in tandem. I discovered that this process systematically revealed the specific problems associated with providing front-line medical care between the Korean War and the later Afghanistan conflict. These included supply problems, indigenous diseases, difficult/austere terrains, and severe changes in climate. I then searched for personal stories of combat medics and individual cases

of casualty survival. Most of the primary text research was obtained from files stored at the UK National Archives, the Imperial War Museum and the Wellcome Unit for the History of Medicine. Further material was found in the US National Archives, New York Public Library, US Air Force Medicine Archives, US Army Medical History Department, the US Navy Bureau of Medical and Surgical Archives, the US Department of Veterans Affairs and in NATO handbooks. I also consulted a whole host of medical journals.

Photographs were mainly obtained from

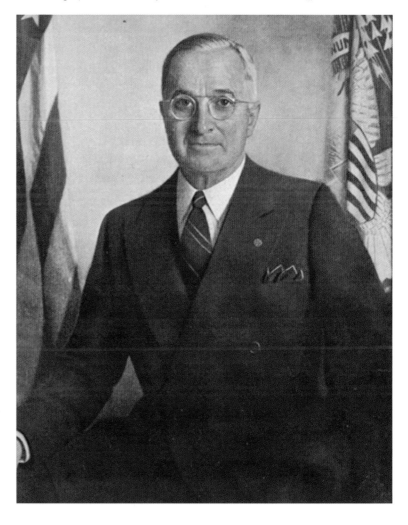

BELOW US President Harry S. Truman. *(New York Public Library, from a painting by Jay Wesley Jacobs)*

the Imperial War Museum, Getty Images, Shutterstock, the Wellcome Unit Photographic Collection, US military websites and the UK Ministry of Defence.

A low point in my research journey came in October 2018 when my father experienced two severe heart attacks. All research trips were placed on hold. This event happened on the same day as my car was in the garage for repair and my computer packed up. They say things happen in threes! Subsequently, I spent some time up in the Midlands helping my father to convalesce. Fortunately, thanks to skilled cardiac surgeons and ITU nurses, plus (I like to think) some aftercare from me his daughter, he recovered well from his cardiac surgery. Moreover, thanks to a University of Bristol computer genius named Raf, my research was back on track by November. The only other hiccup in my research occurred when one of the US websites I had chosen for image research unexpectedly crashed (never to be seen again) leaving me with a lengthy catalogue of reference numbers and no images. The moral of this story

is that I should have downloaded them all at the time of viewing instead of just taking reference numbers… a steep learning curve.

An ongoing problem for most modern historians and researchers centres on the UK National Archives' thirty-year rule preventing viewing of more recent documents. Therefore, much of the archive material relating to the Iraq and Afghanistan conflicts was gleaned from US military archives. Fortunately, however, the UK research gap was later filled by current members of the UK Defence Medical Services. Through the efficient and tireless efforts of Jay Myers, Media Officer at Headquarters Air Command, RAF, I was introduced to a whole host of interesting characters and extremely helpful military medics. These included Wing Commander Bob Tipping and Lieutenant-Colonel Harvey Pynn, who patiently answered all my research queries, provided me with up to date information, and kindly gave me feedback on the first chapter drafts. The information they and others have supplied has received official publication clearance from the Ministry of Defence.

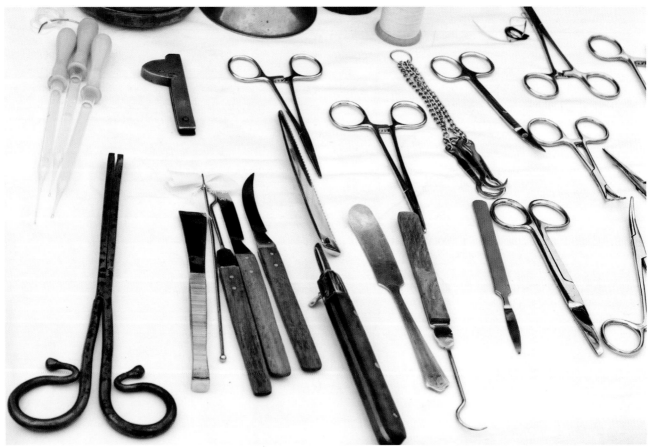

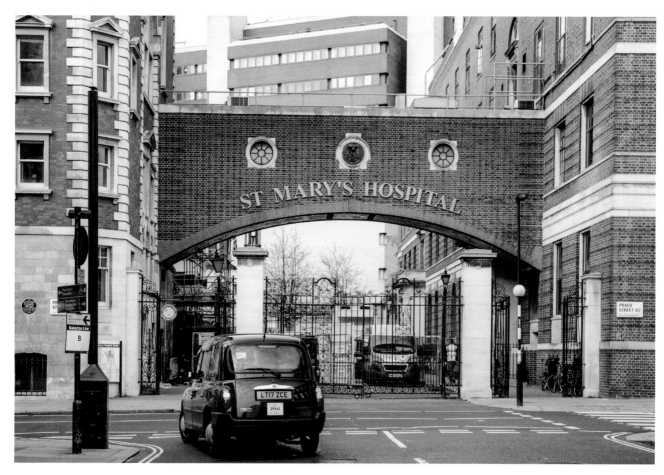

I was surprised by research findings, which revealed some highly unusual and unexpected innovations in the history of combat medicine. For instance, a complex carbohydrate extracted from chitin, the structural component from the shells of crabs and shrimps, has increased blood clotting times and has played a vital role in reducing deaths from haemorrhage. Meanwhile, thanks to phenomenal advances in bio-engineering, the ability to create body integration systems has given hope to thousands of amputees. And moreover, the startling discovery of astroglial scarring in the brain tissue of blast victims offers exciting prospects for new treatments.

But the examination of historical evidence has also revealed a remarkable continuity with the past. Despite major changes in weaponry over the course of a century the aetiology of deaths from battle wounds has remained unchanged. Thus, the proportion of deaths from haemorrhage and traumatic head wounds in later conflicts were not dissimilar to those found on the Western Front in the First World War. Establishing field hospital communities and introducing leisure activities to shore up staff and patient morale were a common feature of all frontline medical units in all wars. The enduring practice of planting flowers, herbs and shrubs around the cold, clinical world of wards and operating theatres, often in the most barren of terrains, also highlighted the abiding human need to focus on life; especially when surrounded by the dead and injured.

Through undertaking extensive research into battlefield medicine, I have come to realise that combat medics provide much more than highly skilled medical care on the frontline of battle. Infused with inspirational courage, a strong sense of duty and stoic tenacity they give their casualties humanitarian, life-affirming hope in situations where it appears that all hope is lost. Crucially, as the Royal Army Medical Corps motto states: they are 'Faithful in Adversity'.

Dr Penny Starns,
Bristol, July 2019.

ABOVE The site in West London of Alexander Fleming's laboratory at St Mary's Hospital, Paddington. *(Shutterstock)*

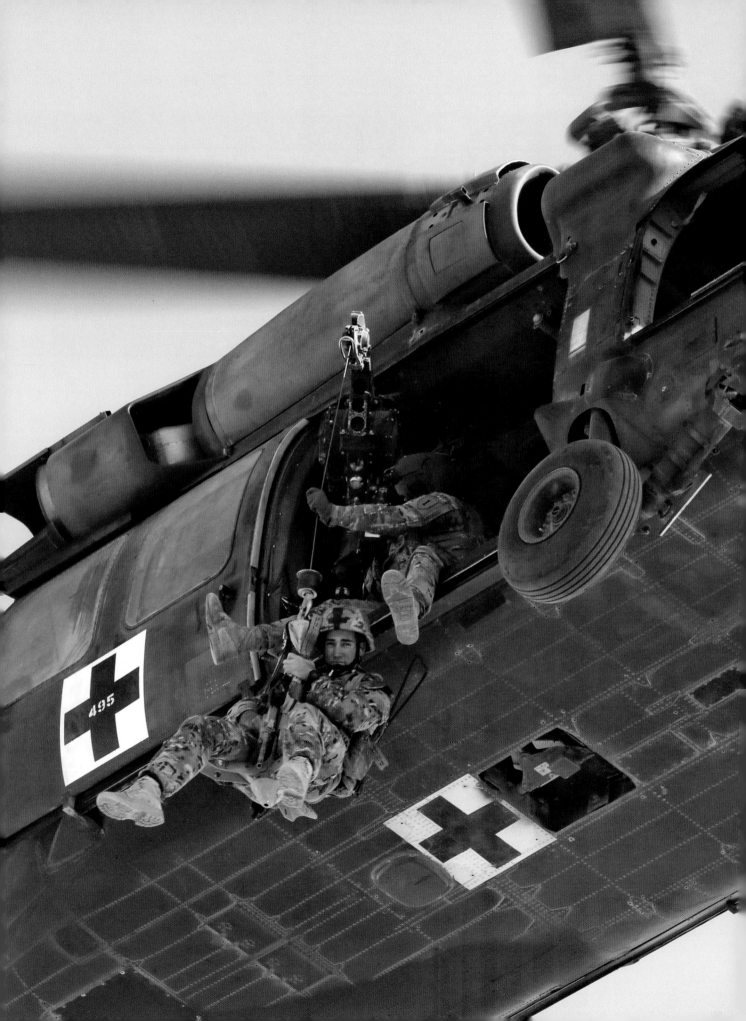

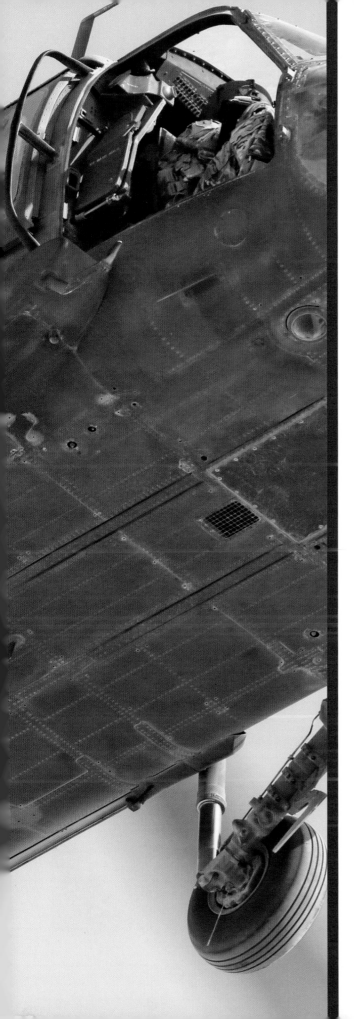

Chapter One

Combat readiness

Preparing military units for combat encompasses a complex range of 'fit for purpose' pre-deployment training exercises. The process of ensuring adequate medical support for fighting forces is equally detailed. In co-operation with NATO allies the UK formulates Clinical Guidelines for Operations. These are dictated by military objectives and strategic considerations.

OPPOSITE A US Army UH-60 Black Hawk helicopter hoists an Australian airman during **MEDEVAC** training on Multinational Base Tarin Kot in Afghanistan's Uruzgan Province, 13 October 2013. *(Australian Defence Force)*

Working on principles established during the Napoleonic Wars, basic structures for ensuring adequate medical support for combat wounded were established by British Director General of Medical Services in the Field, General Arthur Sloggett, in 1916. In preparation for the Somme Offensive, he divided field ambulances into two sections, one placed very near to the front line and the other slightly behind it. It was anticipated that these sections could amalgamate if necessary, to provide large advanced casualty clearing stations. Specialist medical teams, including anaesthetists, orthopaedic and neurological surgeons were placed on call, and makeshift operating theatres were moved to forward areas. Three fully equipped hospital trains were on standby to transport seriously wounded men from casualty clearing stations to base hospitals and further trains were available if required. Sloggett had also ensured that more numbers of medical personnel were on the front line than during previous battles. At 7.30am on 1 July 1916 the Battle of the Somme began; within an hour and a half, 20,000 British soldiers had been killed. By the end of the day there were nearly 60,000 casualties. Front-line field ambulances were completely overwhelmed and overrun with wounded. News of the appalling casualty figures reached Sloggett at 3.00pm and more hospital trains were urgently ordered. However, some of these took over ten hours to reach the Somme.[1]

In fairness to General Sloggett, no one could have predicted the Somme carnage. The positioning of combat medics and casualty clearing stations as near to the front as possible was an excellent, life-saving strategy; and the tiered system of care a well-founded approach. Fundamental medical support arrangements for the Somme, however, had not included a surge capability – effective contingency plans to deal with sudden, enormous and unpredictable increases in casualty numbers. This important lesson from the battlefields of the Western Front was not lost on later generations of military medics.[2]

Undoubtedly the policy of moving medical facilities nearer to the front improved patient outcomes in the Second World War. Moreover, while the Airborne Medical Services experienced initial problems with weight and size limitations, these were eventually overcome by the introduction of specialist equipment. These included the folding airborne stretcher, collapsible wheeled stretcher carriage, light folding trestles, folding suspension bar, airborne operating table, plasma containers for dropping by parachute, insulated blood containers and 'Don' and 'Sugar' packs. The 'Don' packs contain sufficient dressings, drugs, medical comforts, etc, for 20 patients, while the 'Sugar' pack is sufficient for resupply for ten surgical cases in the operating theatre. The methods by which this equipment is taken into action are:

RIGHT Curtiss JN-4 Jenny air ambulance was developed by US Major Nelson E. Driver and Captain William C. Ocker. They successfully modified the open rear cockpit area of a standard JN-4 biplane to receive a stretcher. It was introduced into US Army service on 25 November 1918 and as one of the first air ambulances it displayed the red cross insignia on its fuselage and wings. A scale model of the JN-4 air ambulance hangs in the US Air Force School of Aerospace Medicine in Dayton, Ohio. *(US Air Force photo)*

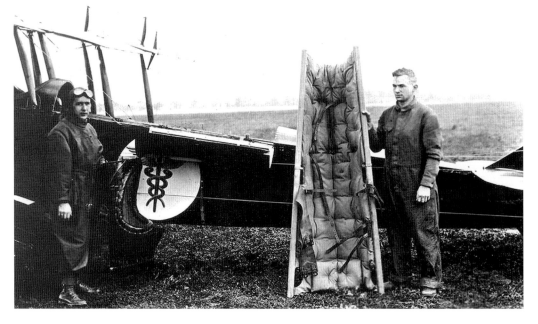

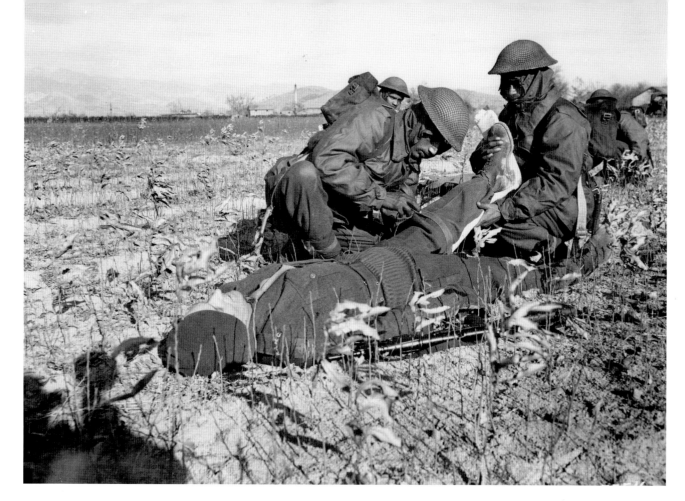

- On the man – in the case of parachute troops, in a kitbag tied to the leg and fitted with a quick release which allows the man to detach the bag from the leg while in the air, the bag then remaining suspended from his belt. In the case of Air Landing Troops, in haversacks or large pack of the web equipment.
- In containers – dropped on parachutes from bomb racks.
- In airborne panniers dropped on parachutes and thrown out of the door of the aircraft.
- In gliders – in this case the medical stores are loaded in jeeps and trailers, and on landing can be conveyed to where they are required.[3]

Although the Director of the British Medical Services issued a prudent warning pertaining to gliders:

Gliders and containers unfortunately do not always land where intended, and it is therefore laid down as a principle in the airborne medical services, that the basic equipment, both for glider and parachute personnel, must be in loads with which the men themselves can land and march. This necessitates the careful selection of essential medical equipment and the packing of it into suitable bundles and packs.[4]

Henceforth aeromedical support became a key feature in determining casualty survival rates, significantly reducing the transport time between point of injury and receiving effective medical treatment. A general trend towards rapid, adaptable mobile medical units pushed surgical teams ever closer to the front line. Yet in the Korean Conflict, despite the proven efficacy of aeromedical evacuations, helicopters were in short supply. A series of budget cuts in the USA seriously curtailed the number of helicopters available to move combat wounded. Senior commanders spoke loudly and publicly of their concern, acknowledging that hundreds of lives were being lost because of this shortage. Hostile terrains and inclement weather also hampered helicopter use. Mobile army surgical hospitals (MASH), were highly successful and naval support for Korean wounded was well organised. Communication networks were also upgraded. However, most

ABOVE Members of the 60th Indian Para Field Ambulance demonstrate first aid during training while on rear echelon duty at Taegu, Korea. This Field Ambulance was divided into two separate entities: one provided medical care to British Commonwealth forces fighting in forward areas, while the other provided medical support to Republic of Korea hospitals at the rear in Taegu. The 60th arrived in Korea in November 1950 and was composed of 346 men, including four combat surgeons, two anaesthetists and a dentist. *(Imperial War Museum – IWM – MH33025)*

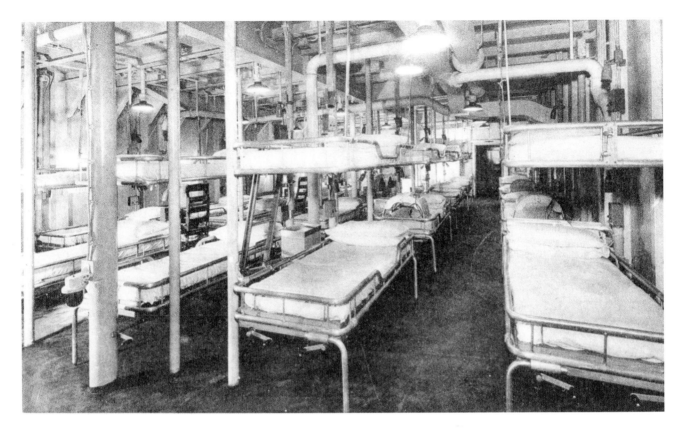

US combat medics only received OJT (on the job training) rather than pre-deployment instruction and preparation.

Medical back-up systems for fighting forces were also frequently hit by supply problems. Occasionally this situation was due to tactical or strategic limitations; times when heavily laden trucks, aircraft or ships could not deliver their goods because it was unsafe to travel through combat zones. US naval nurses insisted that food and medicine shortages were common, because at the beginning of the war no one appeared to have figured out what supplies would be required. With no accurate assessment of possible demands, supplies were quickly depleted when medics received a high volume of casualties. A naval nurse writing in her diary in 1950 on board the USS *Consolation* AH-15 described her work:

4 November 1950 – I live from one crisis to another, and it is 3.30pm before I know it. I go off duty utterly exhausted both physically and mentally. Both a duty and evacuation party are going out tomorrow, and so we must brace ourselves for a fresh onslaught of casualties.

7 November 1950 – What a night! I never stopped running, except for fifteen minutes for dinner. It seems that some sixty Americans met up with a large group of North Koreans and these [casualties] were the survivors. Things couldn't have been any worse. They came in a steady stream [. . .] in shock or next to it. Bloody, dirty and all the rest [. . .] these fellows don't complain. Although two were critical and two serious, we didn't lose them.

9 November 1950 – The doctor told one of my boys [patient], aged twenty, that he would have to lose his right arm. He was running a high temperature, so I tried to combine a few words of comfort with an alcohol rub. But if there is a formula that covers such situations, I haven't found it [. . .] I feel that I have failed miserably.

10 November – Today I hit the jackpot, five letters. Now I understand why even fellows I met just casually used to beg for letters. Mail becomes so terribly important. We are running out of supplies and we leave to go back to Yokosuka.[5]

In Vietnam supply lines were improved, and there were enough helicopters readily available to pick up the wounded from battlefields and transfer them to the nearest care facility. The experience gained in both Korea and Vietnam further demonstrated that within the field of combat medicine, the availability of aeromedical support was crucial in terms of increasing casualty survival rates. Logistical planning for medical support, in or near conflict zones, however, has never been a simple task. Aside from complex tactical, environmental and personnel considerations, planners needed to second guess the enemy, predict likely battle scenarios and mechanisms of injury – and act accordingly.

On occasions logistical decisions have been made based on military medical intelligence. In Vietnam medics initially displayed red cross insignia on their helmets to indicate their status within military units. But this insignia was used by enemy snipers as a moving target and a decision was taken to remove red crosses from helmets and place them on armbands instead. Similarly, when senior medical officers were planning casualty care for the Falklands Campaign, a decision was taken not to display a red cross on the roof of a field hospital at Ajax Bay, nor (at certain times) on hospital ships. Intelligence reports revealed that Argentine forces were aiming to specifically bomb British medical facilities in order to slow down the British advance.[6] Neither did the part-medical ship *Argus*, which was deployed during the Gulf War, display the red cross insignia.

All combat medics wearing the red cross are afforded some protection under the Geneva Convention, and it is a war crime to shoot a medic when he or she is attending to the wounded. This protection is rescinded, however, if medics use firearms to protect their patient, or themselves. But while UK military planners deliberated about when and where this international sign of neutrality could be safely used, the biggest nightmare for US military planners during the conflicts in Iraq was a lack of qualified personnel. Requests for additional staff and resources to meet growing military medical needs were met with stony silence. Consequently, numerous surgeons found

BELOW US Naval Hospital Corps School, USNH Portsmouth, Virginia, Company 120-52, March 1952. This establishment is the oldest US Naval Medical Center and was originally built in 1827. *(US Navy photo)*

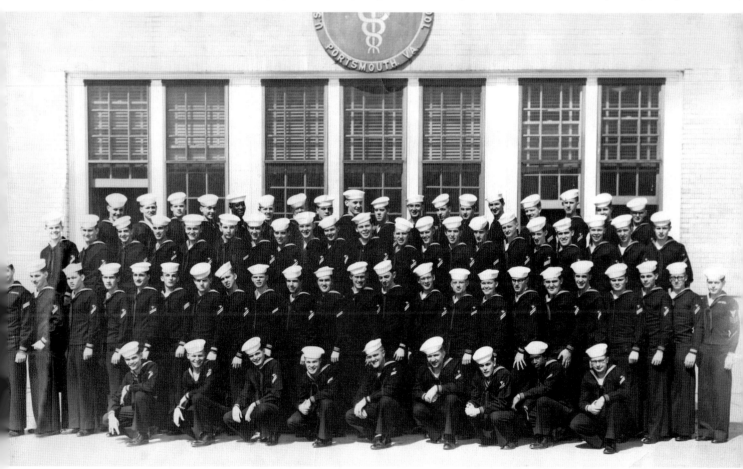

themselves on extended, second and third deployments. Even this policy was not enough to fill the gap and specialist surgeons were commandeered to assume the role of general surgeons.

Logistical situations such as these were not a new occurrence. Problems associated with either personnel, transport, equipment or supply problems have featured in most wars, but the fundamental tiered approach to providing casualty care has changed little since 1916. For the USA and members of the North Atlantic Treaty Organization (NATO), multinational, multidisciplinary, military medical support procedures are divided into four levels of care described as roles or echelons. Army and air force personnel usually refer to care levels as roles, whereas maritime forces tend to use the term echelon. Both are defined according to medical capabilities and resources. Casualties do not have to progress through each echelon in order to receive care, ie they can be seen by medics at any level depending on their needs.

■ Role one – these medical aid stations are staffed by combat medics, doctors and/or doctors' assistants. They provide basic first aid point-of-injury care, or care at a battalion aid station. Treatment is limited but basic triage can occur.

■ Role two – these medical units can provide basic and advanced emergency treatment; they contain blood supplies, laboratory facilities, X-ray imaging and other medical support such as dentistry, physiotherapy and occupational therapy. Some even provide combat stress counselling. This level of care also has a patient holding capacity, with or without critical care facilities. Within modern battle space scenarios these units are often boosted with a forward surgical team (FST), thus elevating them into two-plus roles. Usually located in the same area, these teams, working together, can perform damage-control surgery, and provide forward surgical treatment for casualties who are not stable enough to be transported elsewhere.

■ Role three – these are larger medical support establishments such as combat support field hospitals. With a capacity of 248 beds or more, such facilities provide most of the treatments associated with modern civilian hospitals. Offering damage-control surgery and definitive-repair surgery, they usually include vascular and thoracic specialists, neurosurgeons and general surgeons, in addition to orthopaedic and trauma specialists.

■ Role four – these are fully equipped and staffed static hospitals which are usually located away from active battle zones. They provide all medical and surgical treatments commonly associated with modern hospitals. Often these hospitals are based in the casualty's country of origin.[7]

In 2006 combat support hospitals (CSH) replaced MASH units. FSTs now move directly behind troops and can erect a field hospital with combat support medical facilities within an hour. They have enough equipment to establish a fully operational hospital as near to the front line as possible. Deployable Rapid Assembly Shelter tents can also be interconnected to make a 900ft^2 care facility. There are enough supplies to resuscitate and operate on the wounded, with intensive care packs, general and orthopaedic surgery packs, anaesthesia and theatre technician packs, anaesthesia apparatus, sterile surgical instruments, operating theatre gowns and curtains, catheters and medicines, plus small units for measuring blood gases and electrolytes. Among FST resources are transportable ventilators, oxygen, monitors, portable ultrasound machines and a plentiful supply of blood. They have enough supplies to examine combat wounded and operate on the injured if necessary. An FST has at least two operating tables, with ventilator-equipped beds to provide initial post-operative critical care.

Moreover, within CSHs scenes of appalling injuries are an everyday occurrence. US Navy Captain Michael McCarten spent a year (2010–11) commanding NATO Role-three Multinational Medical Unit in Kandahar. Writing in 2011 he described his experiences:

Medics roll a badly wounded US soldier into the military hospital in Kandahar, Afghanistan. He has lost both his legs to a roadside bomb, and his head and neck are torn up. The international surgical team snaps into action to clean his exposed flesh; specialists

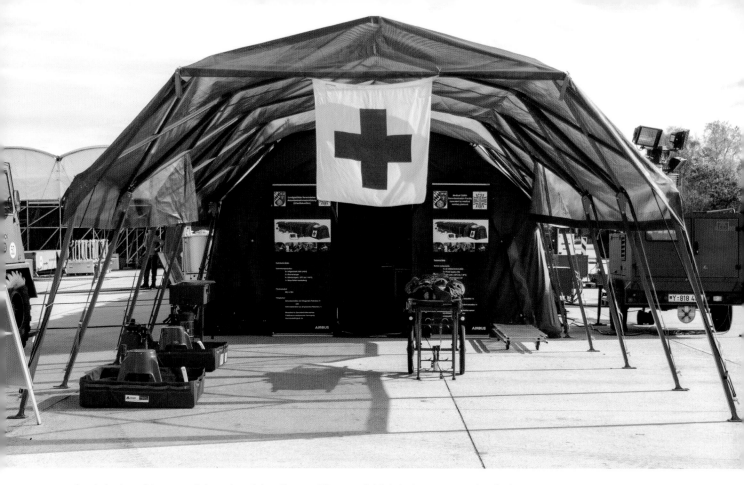

check for head trauma. A few days later, the bandaged young soldier is flown to another military hospital for more surgery, then begins his journey home to recover. The trauma we see here is devastating. Sometimes the anatomy is unrecognizable.[8]

The crucial link between every level of casualty care within NATO nomenclatures is aeromedical support. Ground vehicles are only used to evacuate casualties when there is a shortage of aeromedical resources; or in cases where aeromedical support is grounded

ABOVE German Military Field Hospital during a medical evaluation exercise at Münster, Germany, on 9 October 2017. Münster was also the location of the post-war British Military Hospital (St Luke's), which finally closed its doors in 1991. *(Shutterstock)*

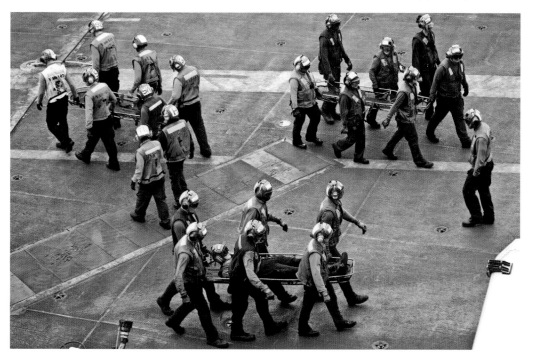

LEFT Flight deck personnel carry stretchers during a mass casualty drill on board the nuclear-powered supercarrier USS *Nimitz* in the Pacific Ocean, 6 May 2013. *(Getty Images)*

due to poor weather conditions or tactical limitations. Ground vehicles are specially adapted ambulance-type vehicles with a medic on board. If a non-medical vehicle or aircraft is used to transport casualties it is termed as a casualty evacuation or Casevac; and at this level very little or no medical care is administered to casualties en route to Roles one to three. In cases where combat medics or nurses are on hand to provide emergency resuscitative treatment en route to care facilities, the casualty evacuation is termed as a medical evacuation or MEDEVAC. These casualties tend to be transported via medically equipped helicopters. Advanced levels of aeromedical care are provided by teams of critical care medics, nurses and technicians in specially equipped and adapted fixed-wing aircraft. The standard

critical care team consists of a consultant anaesthetist, anaesthetic registrar, two ICU nurses, a medical assistant (flight medic) and an equipment technician. This team may be further augmented depending on requirement.[9]

NATO principles of medical support for operational planning are divided into twenty-three sections. Significantly they state:

Medical resources in theatre must be designed to provide from the onset of the mission, sufficient capabilities to adequately provide all levels of support. Medical support must expand progressively as force strength expands and risks increase and should have a surge capability to deal with peak casualty rates in excess of expected daily rates, understanding that the peaks will be beyond the capability to provide normal care.[10]

BELOW German Army personnel assigned to Kabul Multinational Brigade hospital in Afghanistan practise patient on and off-loading procedures on a US Army HH-60 Blackhawk helicopter, 14 January 2003. *(Getty Images)*

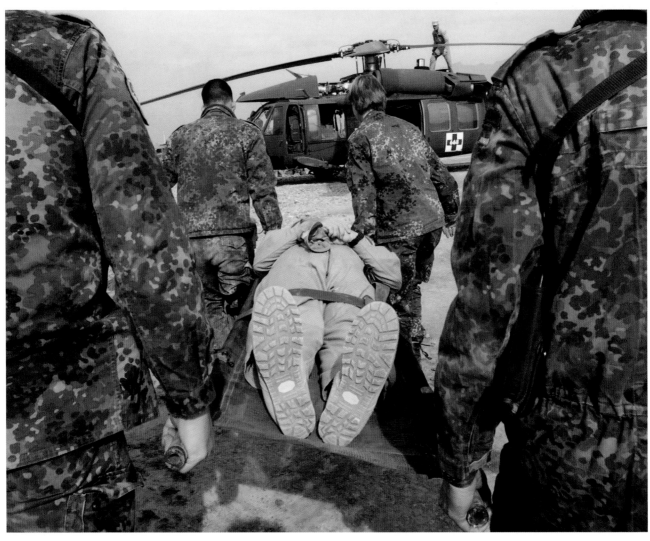

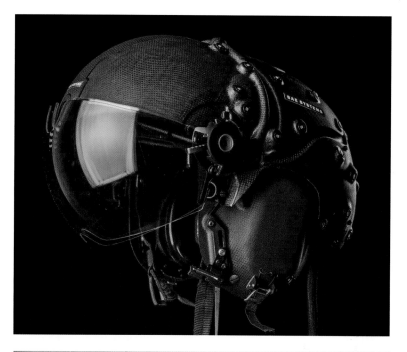

In addition to the overall logistics of tactical combat casualty care, NATO also stresses the importance of personnel preparation. Therefore, armed forces in all NATO countries ensure that military personnel are fully combat ready before deployment. Extremely high standards of health and fitness levels are required for all members of the military and these are regularly assessed. Personnel are given protective combat clothing and equipment prior to deployment and inoculations are administered to maintain fighting strength in the field. Both methods of combat and environmental factors influence these measures. Protective body- and headgear are provided for troops, and specialised helmets for fighter pilots. A wide variety of armoured vehicles, including ships, mine-resistant, ambush-protected personnel carriers and sophisticated aircraft, defend against mortar fire and other missiles.

Inoculations, meanwhile, are formulated to protect against disease and are usually dictated by tactical mission environments and medical intelligence. For example, a lack of clean water, hot humid conditions and poor hygiene standards in Vietnam prompted numerous outbreaks of diarrhoea. Thousands of troops suffered from mild bouts of intestinal illness, but cholera inoculations were successful. Despite several cholera epidemics in Vietnam, the herd immunity prevented troops from contracting

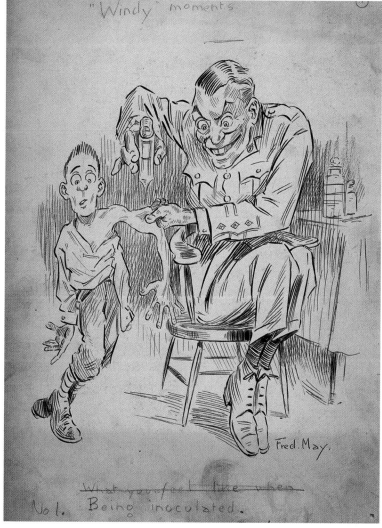

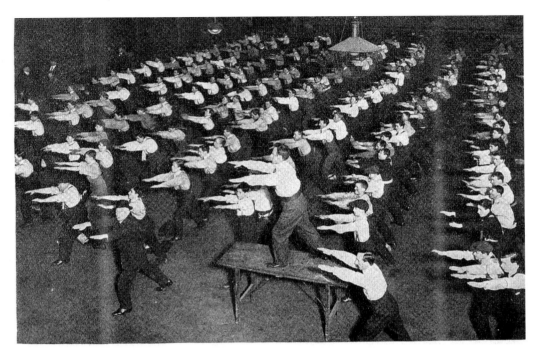

the disease. Nonetheless, it was impossible to inoculate against all disease and a rare Pseudomonas strain emerged in the 1960s causing meliodosis in soldiers. There were 30 cases in 1966 and almost a third of these died. Prophylactic use of drugs was also used to protect against disease. In Vietnam, during a period of five years, over 40,000 soldiers contracted malaria and 78 of these men died. Anti-malaria Amodioquine (Camoquin) tablets were used to protect troops, but in the 1980s severe side effects, such as toxic hepatitis, were reported. This condition fatally lowered immunity

levels and the product was withdrawn. Some inoculations have since proved controversial. For instance, immunisations against biological warfare, combined with pyridostigmine bromide (anti-nerve agent tablets), administered to military personnel prior to their deployment in the First Gulf War, was initially implicated in 'Gulf War Syndrome'.

Along with physical preparation for combat, military personnel are equipped psychologically for war. Respect for leadership, unit cohesion, high morale, positive attitudes and mental alertness are all features of psychological training. For combat medics this training has an added dimension; keeping cool under pressure and making quick decisions are essential mental characteristics for saving lives on the battlefield. Given the phenomenal pressure of tending to the wounded under fire, mental focus is crucial. Stress inoculation training (SIT) which 'reduces arousal levels in response to powerful stressors by "inoculating" individuals to potentially traumatizing stressors, works on the premise that: stress occurs when the perceived demands of a situation exceed an individual's ability to cope. This is particularly acute when stressors are uncontrollable or unpredictable.'[11] This is essential, owing to the chaotic, turbulent situations which combat medics deal with on a regular basis.

Confronting emotionally disturbing scenes of

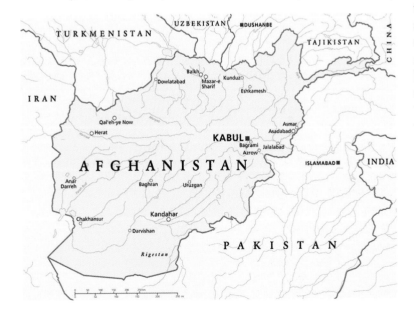

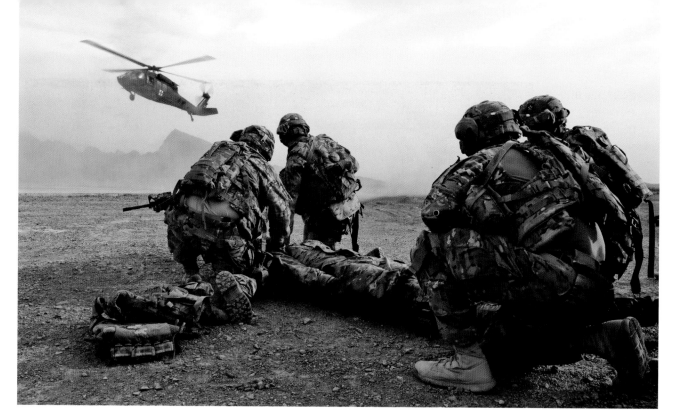

severely mutilated men, hearing their screams of agonising pain and performing skilled medical procedures while dodging bullets and mortar fire is no mean feat. In a battlefield scenario where everything happens all at once, a combat medic needs to prioritise medical emergencies. High standards of pre-deployment training are crucial to assist medics in keeping a cool head under pressure. Studies conducted at the US Army Research Laboratory before troop deployment to Iraq suggested that virtual reality simulators were highly efficient in improving decision-making and enhancing practical skills in combat scenarios.

Those trained in simulation while having stressors added (being shot at while attending to wounded) were able to perform skills more effectively in the test phase of the study compared to those trained in a 'sterile' virtual environment (with no shooting). Those receiving SIT were able to develop divided attention skills and learned to moderate physiological responses to stress while staying focussed on the task at hand. Those not receiving SIT were pulled off task and experienced much more physical arousal during the test phase (being shot at), which caused mistakes to be made (simulated patients died, or medics were killed in action).[12]

Following on from initial successes associated with simulation training, innovative equipment has been produced which mimics the appearance, noise and atmosphere of combat zones. Practical medical and surgical skills are enhanced using specialist haemostatic and multiple amputation trainers. At the Royal College of Surgeons in the UK, military operational surgical courses are situated in a special simulation suite. Scenarios have been designed to reflect current practice in the field in Afghanistan.[13] Meanwhile, Army Medical Services offer HOSPEX courses, where aircraft hangars are mocked up to resemble field hospitals with all available personnel and equipment being present. In order to provide a fully immersive experience, candidates dress in the same clothing that they would wear on deployment, including body armour CS95 clothing and desert boots.[14] Simulation exercises involving practical medical skills and evacuation procedures are practised both pre-deployment and during deployment. Furthermore, it is important to recognise from the outset that military medical training is dramatically different to civilian training. Aside from variations between military and civilian equipment and medical protocols, patterns of injury differ considerably in operational settings. As Consultant Anaesthetist Simon Mercer has pointed out: 'The military hospital

ABOVE Provincial Reconstruction Team security force members wait for a UH-60 Blackhawk medevac helicopter to land before moving a simulated casualty during medical training, Afghanistan, 9 January 2013. *(US Navy photo)*

in Iraq and currently in Afghanistan manages much more severe trauma than an average UK hospital.' Alarm signals also differ: 'In a conflict environment, an alarm bell ringing may signify the need to drop down flat on the floor ('on your belt buckle') to protect you from an incoming mortar attack. This is different from the NHS where it might signify a fire alarm or the cardiac arrest bleep.'[15]

For some, the difference between civilian and military trauma care amounted to a baptism of fire; as highlighted by Squadron Leader Charlotte Thompson-Edgar ARRC, who described her nursing experiences when rescuing injured personnel in Afghanistan:

There was no training for the job, and I had never done any pre-hospital care. I was used to working in a nice emergency room in a safe environment with kit and everyone on standby. Suddenly I was in a Chinook helicopter, unable to hear myself think, treating guys with horrific injuries and being shot at. I was not prepared to see these injuries but then the military was not

expecting to see them either. I pulled 600 patients from the battlefield – about 80% of them had limbs missing or gunshot wounds. Quite a lot died, especially those with gunshot wounds to the head and chest. We also saw guys who were dying because they were losing too much blood.[16]

As a result of her encounters with combat trauma, Thompson-Edgar resolved to ensure that other medics were better prepared for the battlefield. Once back in the UK, she enlisted the help of amputee soldiers to establish a new Medical Emergency Response Team (MERT) training programme. This pre-deployment training enabled medics to gain vital instruction in dealing with real amputees and acquire a greater understanding of tactical combat casualty care.

Medics also learn basic survival techniques. Within maritime environments, courses include instructions on methods of firefighting, chemical, biological, radiological, nuclear (CBRN) courses, damage repair instructional units (DRIU), basic sea survival courses and helicopter ditching

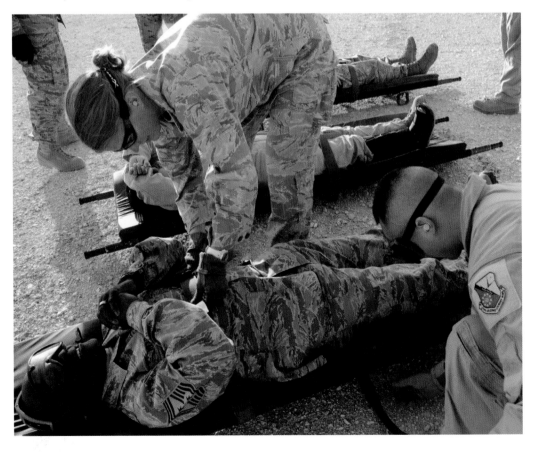

RIGHT A Critical Care Aeromedical Transport Team (CCATT) conduct a demonstration. In addition to practising critical care procedures, the teams also test the safety and efficacy of intensive care equipment. *(US Air Force photo)*

escape training. Aeromedical Critical Care Air Support (CCAST) team members undergo regular equipment instruction and train in simulated environments such as a Hercules Rear Crew Trainer and a Chinook simulator.

Saving lives in combat zones clearly depends on the speedy application of medical knowledge, and it makes sense to train every combatant in basic first aid. First response preparation includes detailed instructions on the rapid assessment of tactical environmental safety issues and casualty needs. Training encompasses the principles of triage, tourniquet application, the best method of performing cardiopulmonary resuscitation (CPR), how to obtain intravenous and intraosseous vascular access, methods of administering fluids and controlling pain, principles of maintaining a clear airway and treatment techniques for tension pneumothorax, how to deal with head, face, eye, torso and limb injuries, plus the management of burns and hypothermia. Effective communication skills are also crucial. Self-aid and buddy care is widely taught and is effective both in terms of saving lives and maintaining morale. This was highlighted during the Falklands Campaign, when no wounded man who was picked up alive died of his wounds. Though a surgeon instructing combatants wryly recalled: 'On a lighter note it may be mentioned the readiness of parachutists to volunteer their brethren-in-arms for training in rectal infusions.'[17]

In recent years pre-deployment training has been standardised across NATO forces, encouraging a multidisciplinary approach to combat medicine. This approach has significantly improved casualty survival rates. Recognising that catastrophic haemorrhage is the number one cause of combat fatalities, training reflects the need to prioritise this condition. The military resuscitation algorithm is:

<C> ABC

Contemporary training therefore focuses on controlling *catastrophic haemorrhage* before proceeding to care for *airway*, *breathing* and *circulation*. Furthermore, this is the most important lesson from the battlefield to be adopted by civilian trauma centres.[18]

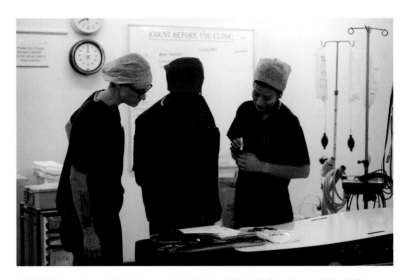

ABOVE A partnership between the National Health Service and the US Air Force's 48th Medical Group based at RAF Lakenheath in Suffolk allows the 48th to maintain readiness in trauma care and battlefield medicine. *(US Air Force photo)*

According to the US Defense Department, current character traits required for the modern combat medic are: an ability to communicate effectively, an ability to work under stressful conditions, a desire to help people and meticulous attention to detail. Undertaking instruction courses which are far removed from the 1950s on-the-job training of Korean War medics, US Army medics are known as the 68W. This reflects their 68 weeks of training. All recruits are required to score at least 101 when taking the Army Service Vocational Aptitude Battery (ASVAB), which consists of a series of multiple-choice tests designed to determine aptitude for vacancies. This score is high compared to the score of 31 required for regular enlistment. Once recruits for the 68W course are accepted, they attend basic military training followed by advanced medical training. This includes emergency medical techniques, advanced medical care and plaster casting techniques.[19]

Each NATO country has its own criteria for admission and instruction courses, but pre-deployment standardised training programmes have impacted favourably on patient outcomes. Crucially, however, military training for combat medics continues to evolve in response to changes in weaponry, mechanisms of injury, lessons from the battlefield and evidence-based research studies.

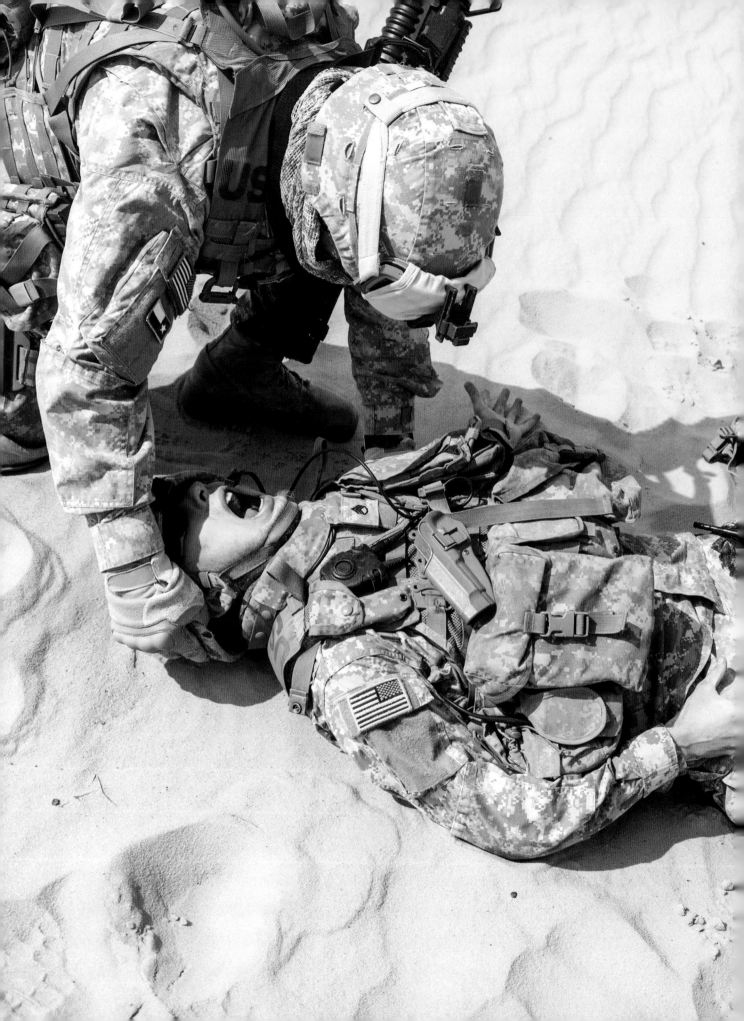

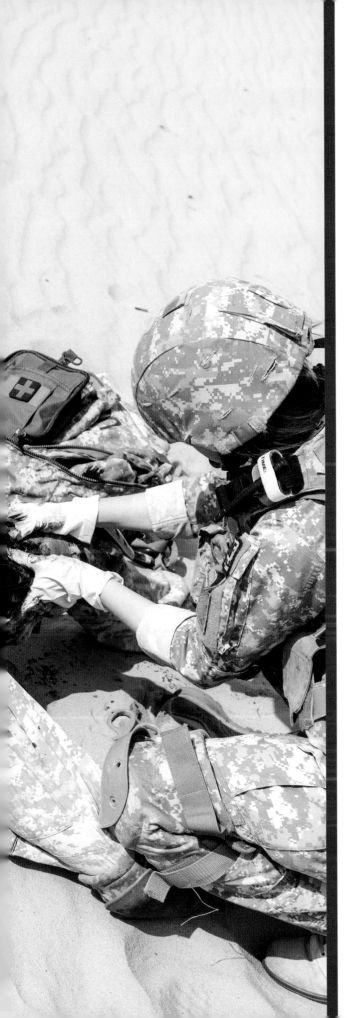

Chapter Two

First response

First response combat medics
provide front-line casualty care
at the point of injury. They adhere
to the 'platinum ten minutes'
rule, which states that decisions
taken, and medical treatment
given within this time frame largely
determines casualty survival rates.

**OPPOSITE Battlefield first aid to a bleeding leg wound.
Injuries to lower limbs are common in combat zones where the
treatment priority is to prevent haemorrhage, clean exposed
tissue and immobilise fractures.** *(Shutterstock)*

RESUSCITATION CHART

D — DANGER

Use all senses to check for dangers to yourself, others and the patient. Ensure the area is safe. Move the patient only if the danger cannot be eliminated.

R — RESPONSE

Check for a normal response by talking to the patient, asking them their name and squeezing their shoulders
DO NOT move the patient if the injury is the result of a fall

S — SEND FOR HELP

Send a bystander to call for help and an Ambulance as soon as possible

DIAL 000 and ask for Ambulance attendance.

A — AIRWAY

Open mouth and check for foreign objects. If objects are present place in recovery position and clear airway with fingers.
DO NOT move patient if the injury is the result of a fall.

B — BREATHING

Check breathing. **Look** for rise and fall of chest. **Listen** for breathing sounds. **Feel** for breaths on the cheek and for ribcage movement. If breathing is present keep the patient in the recovery position and monitor.

C — CPR

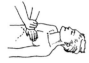

If no breathing is present commence CPR.
Give 30 Chest Compressions to every 2 Breaths @ 100 Compressions/minute.

D — DEFIBRILLATION

AED

Apply defibrillator (if available) and follow the voice prompts or instruction on the device.
AED - Automated External Defibrillator

Continue CPR until responsiveness or normal breathing returns

FIRE & SAFETY AUSTRALIA

www.fsaus.com.au | 1300 88 55 30
www.nsca.org.au | 1800 65 55 10

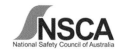
National Safety Council of Australia

The purpose of combat medics is to save lives and alleviate suffering on the battlefield. In order to do their work, they need to be well trained, quick thinking and clear headed. In theory, they are also taught to protect themselves first, before going to the aid of others. In practice, however, combat medics frequently put their own lives on the line while attending to the injured. All soldiers, sailors and airmen are taught the principles of self-aid and buddy care. They all carry mission-dependent first-aid packs. But only combat medics can perform advanced medical skills such as obtaining vascular access by means of intravenous or intraosseous intervention.

In Korea and Vietnam emphasis was placed on delivering front-line medical care within a 'golden hour'. This 60-minute time-frame was measured from point-of-injury sites to admission to care facilities. Any delay beyond this point largely determined casualty survival rates. In recent years lessons from combat zones have shifted this emphasis towards medical aid given within a platinum ten minutes. Furthermore,

whereas military first-aid doctrine used to follow the ABC rule – airway, breathing and circulation – the number of lives lost on battlefields because of catastrophic haemorrhage highlighted the need to stem uncontrolled bleeding before attending to airways. Therefore, the current rule is < C > ABC, the first 'C' denoting that preventing catastrophic haemorrhage is the priority. In Vietnam, nearly 3,000 troops died from extremity haemorrhage, and it remains the leading cause of battlefield deaths to this day.

To some extent all injured personnel experience a complex condition known as shock. Severe blood loss, penetrating wounds, brain and blast injuries are just some of its causes. Field medics are taught to treat all wounded as though they are suffering, or about to suffer, from shock. This is because signs such as skin colour (deathly pale or grey), tachycardia, collapsed veins, a lack of peripheral perfusion and extreme cold (unless shivering is present) may be difficult to detect on the battlefield. In severe cases it is

OPPOSITE
Resuscitation diagram.

BELOW A wounded British lieutenant receives aid from a US 3rd Infantry Division medic near Ui jong-bu, Korea. The 3rd became renowned for its quick response on the battlefield and was awarded ten battle stars at the end of the conflict. *(IWM KOR659)*

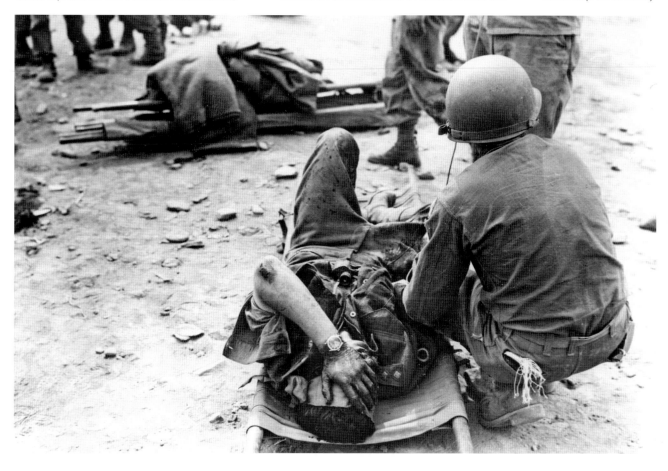

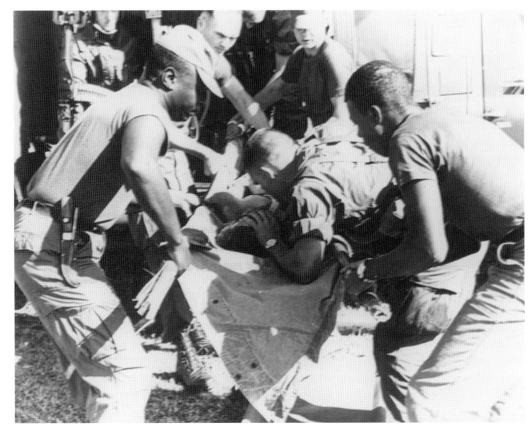

impossible to feel a pulse of any description. Sufferers have physically 'shut down'. When a body enters a state of shock it reduces blood flow to peripheral blood vessels to conserve oxygenated blood supplies for vital organs, such as the brain and heart. Simultaneously the body activates clotting mechanisms, but this is futile when arterial blood is gushing out of the body. In cases of haemorrhagic shock, this process happens very quickly. If blood loss persists, the heart works even harder and faster to pump remaining blood to organs, the body becomes hypothermic and metabolic acidosis (leaking of acid from oxygenated blood-starved organs) occurs. By this stage sufferers experience respiratory distress and their chances of survival are minimal. It is vital therefore that shock is either prevented, or, if present, treated as a matter of urgency. Arresting haemorrhage, keeping sufferers warm and initiating fluid resuscitation is a life-saving protocol of treatment.

However, as the first to arrive on the scene, and before any first aid can be administered, a medic needs to gauge the overall situation. Scenarios of care are roughly divided into three sections: care under fire, tactical field care (when firing has ceased but medic and casualty are still in the conflict zone) and tactical evacuation care. During the first two scenarios medical equipment is limited and casualty management variable. When under fire, if possible, casualties are moved to a safe covered area. Measures are then put in place to protect existing casualties from sustaining further injury and to prevent more casualties. If ground cover or shelter is not available, the wounded are instructed to lie flat while a medic issues instruction for self-aid. The nature of tactical missions, availability of equipment and night-time visual limitations may prevent medics from examining the wounded thoroughly in the first instance; but life-threatening blood loss is treated immediately. For bleeding limbs, tourniquets can be quickly self-applied by the casualty, high on the extremity and over clothing. The limb is then elevated if possible. When applied before the onset of shock, chances of survival are greatly improved. If bleeding persists then a second tourniquet is applied slightly higher on the limb than the first device. It requires three revolutions of the

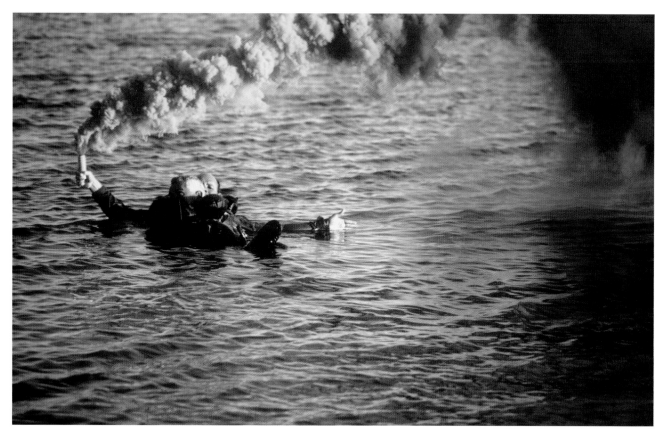

ABOVE Rescue at sea, waiting for help. Those injured at sea often suffer from severe hypothermia. However, the high concentration of salt in sea water is beneficial to the healing of open wounds. *(Getty Images)*

windlass to stall bleeding, and the distal pulse is assessed to ensure bleeding has stopped.

Tourniquets fell out of favour in the 1950s and '60s and became the subject of much controversy. Medical opinion was divided between those who advocated their use as a life-saving device, and those who believed they did more harm than good. The latter group argued that misapplication and prolonged use irreparably damaged limbs that could have been salvaged. Faced with a lack of statistical data, the controversy dragged on for decades. Certainly, tourniquets left in place for longer than

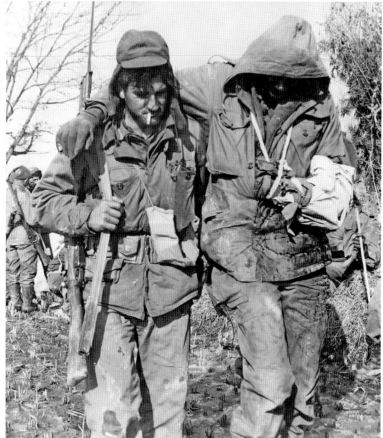

RIGHT Soldier helping his wounded comrade in Korea. All military personnel were taught basic first aid and the importance of attending to injured members of their unit. *(IWM BF427)*

two hours did put limbs at risk of permanent ischaemia and nerve damage, resulting in higher amputation rates. During the Vietnam War tourniquets were only intermittently carried by field medics, although some improvised by using belts or ropes to stem bleeding. Applications of tourniquets and possible limb salvage largely depended on casualty evacuation times. If evacuation was delayed, then limb damage was often unavoidable, though orthopaedic surgeons were quick to acknowledge that it was better for soldiers to lose a limb rather than their lives.

In recent conflicts, however, there has been a resurgence of tourniquet use. In Iraq, a study of 499 US soldiers showed beyond any doubt that these devices saved lives. Further statistical evidence confirmed these findings. As a result, tourniquets are a mandatory addition to the first-aid packs of all members of US military and NATO coalition forces. They are also attached to a soldier's uniform with Velcro and designed for easy single-handed application. Although straightforward and cost-effective, complications of tourniquet use include acidosis, reduced limb temperature, low tissue oxygen, the accumulation of carbon dioxide and nerve injury. However, standard-issue devices and rigorous training in appropriate applications have successfully overcome these drawbacks. Moreover, when correctly applied, combat application tourniquets (CATs) can be safely left in situ for two hours before any permanent tissue, nerve and blood vessel damage is caused. They are usually left in position until the casualty is evacuated. In circumstances where evacuation time is likely to be over two hours, medics establish fluid resuscitation before tourniquets are slackened, and haemorrhage is controlled by other means. In combat environments, applying compression to non-extremity wounds is extremely problematic, especially if working under fire. Direct pressure is sometimes effective but difficult to maintain. Such wounds usually require urgent surgical intervention, in tactical field care they can be treated with haemostatic dressings and drugs once casualties have been moved to a place of safety. Junctional tourniquets are also effective if available and used appropriately.

COMPARISON OF JUNCTIONAL TOURNIQUETS

	Combat ready clamp	Junctional emergency	Junctional tourniquets
mechanism	Mechanical	Mechanical	Pneumatic
FDA-approved regions of application	Delto-pectoral groove Groin (unilateral) Neck (as a last resort for significant carotid artery bleeding) Umbilicus (as a last resort for significant bilateral bleeding not controllable by any other method)	Groin*	Delto-pectoral groove Groin*
Vessel occluded	Axillary artery Common femoral artery Carotid artery Aortic bifurcation	Common femoral artery	Axillary artery Common femoral artery
Notes	Unilateral use	Bilateral use (for groin) Literature supports use as pelvic stabiliser	Bilateral use (for groin)

Notes: FDA: US Food and Drug Administration
*Device used for bilateral occlusion of bleeding from both groins
(Source: R. Chang, B.J. Eastridge and J.B. Holcombe, 'Tactical Combat Casualty Care: Transitioning Battlefield Lessons Learned to other Austere Environments', *Wilderness and Environmental Medicine*, 28 (2017), S124–S134.

Often in the middle of nowhere, deafened by hostile bomb blasts and gunfire, surrounded by mutilated blood-splattered bodies, medics must make a choice of whose wounds to treat first. Whether conducted on the battlefield, in transit or in hospital corridors, triage is a vital part of a medic's job. Confronted with multiple casualties, their instinct is to prioritise those who are badly wounded. But in instances where resources are limited, and time is of the essence, this is not always the wisest option, as Dr Rick Jolly asserted when faced with overwhelming casualty numbers after the bombing of RFA *Sir Galahad* in 1982:

As darkness crept over the horizon, load after load of helicopter casualties began to arrive at Ajax Bay. Each new patient seemed worse than the last; eventually the triage and resuscitation areas were choked. Helicopters continued to clatter in, and stretcher-borne casualties kept appearing at the main door [. . .] In the demanding circumstances of a Mass Casualty Situation, the normal principles of priority for medical treatment get completely inverted. With normal casualty loadings, you tackle the most severely injured first, while the least injured have to wait. That instinctive reaction had to be suppressed now. Instead, we had to do the best we could for the largest number and recognise that some of our potential customers might be too badly injured to treat – because they would take up too much in the way of time and resources, and thereby reduce the chance of others.[1]

Faced with floods of injured personnel triage is, of necessity, ruthless: 'Triage is a dynamic business, and priorities for waiting cases can change constantly. The triage officer has to be a sharp, totally aware cookie.'[2]

Instructions for giving care to the wounded when under fire, therefore, are to avoid engaging in pointless resuscitation efforts. When both medics and casualties are under fire, CPR is usually only given to victims of drowning or electrocution, or to those suffering from hypothermia. Attempts to perform CPR on blast victims who have no pulse or other vital signs of life are often a lost cause and expose medics to bullets and rocket fire. Furthermore, time spent trying to resuscitate those without hope of recovery means that medical attention is withheld from those who have a better chance of survival. Airway management of patients is also normally withheld until the tactical field care phase.

Although urgent care is often given under fire, once the injured are sheltered by ground cover, plucked from the battlefield by rescue helicopters or when hostile fire has ceased, medical care can be given unhindered. Within the platinum ten minutes medics need to assess patients for the following:

- shock and blood loss
- neurogenic shock (spinal injury)
- anaphylactic shock
- control of external bleeding
- soft tissue injuries
- fractures and dislocations
- skull fractures
- brain injuries
- facial injuries
- spinal injuries
- abdominal injuries
- genitalia injuries.[3]

When bleeding is under control, airway management is the next consideration. No intervention is required if the casualty is conscious and breathing adequately; but if unconscious a clear airway can usually be maintained by a simple chin lift. The casualty is then placed in the recovery position to prevent inhalation of stomach contents, blood or mucus. If an airway is necessary, in terms of ease and stability a nasopharyngeal airway is preferred over an oropharyngeal device. In cases of severe blunt trauma, it is important to immobilise the cervical spine. If airway obstruction is caused by face and neck injuries, and it is impossible to see the vocal cords clearly, a cricothyroidotomy is required.

Casualties struggling to breathe on the battle field are most likely to have sustained penetrating chest wounds or severe trauma to the torso. These can produce tension pneumothorax. Victims of such injuries have a build-up of air within the pleural cavity which shifts the mediastinum and obstructs venous return to

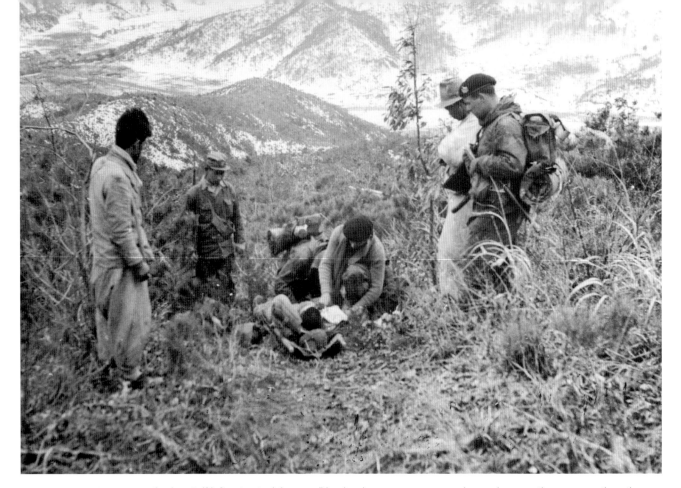

ABOVE A Chinese soldier receives medical attention in Korea by his captors from the 1st Battalion Gloucestershire Regiment. During the Battle of Imjin River in April 1951, 650 soldiers of the 'Glorious Glosters' fought off 10,000 Chinese troops. This action gave remaining United Nations (UN) forces a chance to regroup and prevent the communist advance on Seoul.
(IWM BF382)

the heart. If left untreated the condition leads to shock, cardiac arrest and death. In civilian hospitals medics are taught to detect signs of tension pneumothorax by observing tracheal shift, hyper-resonance on percussion and changes in breath sounds. Combat medics, however, are taught to assume the worst. There is no room for subtlety on the battlefield. Open chest wounds are covered with occlusive chest seals during expiration; while tension pneumothorax is treated with needle decompression. A 14- to 16-gauge needle catheter is inserted into an intercostal space. The needle is then removed, leaving the catheter buried to the hub. Subsequent monitoring of the patient is important, because occasionally the catheter becomes displaced or obstructed by blood clots. If this occurs, a second needle catheter is inserted next to the first. Haemothorax and pleural effusions, lung contusions and a variety of breathing problems can be caused by battlefield injuries. These are not always immediately obvious. A lieutenant in Korea described his experience of lung complications:

> The Chinese apparently had illuminating grenades. They would work their way closer to our lines . . . throw several illuminating grenades and survey the area . . . then throw offensive concussion grenades and move forward. The effect was eerie, with a yellow-white light reflecting off the snow, and the Chinese looked ghostlike in their white parka uniforms. The explosions were all around me. I felt a sting in my left leg but otherwise I was lucky. We stopped them briefly, but they regrouped and came on again. This time I wasn't so lucky. I was hit hard in the arm, wrist and chest by [shrapnel from] two or three grenades. I crawled back to the Command Post to get a bandage on my wrist, which was bleeding profusely. The corpsman bandaged my wrist. I started back up the hill but discovered I had great difficulty walking. I didn't think my wrist would cause all that difficulty. What I did not know at the time was that I had two pieces of shrapnel in my chest, my lung was collapsed, and my chest filled with fluid. Try as I might, I just couldn't function. So, I sat down again and asked the corpsman if he could do anything. He said there was an aid station just down the trail. They could get me there. I staggered and stumbled to the aid station [. . .] and spent two days at a field hospital during heavy attacks.[4]

GLASGOW COMA SCALE

Behaviour	Response	Score
Eye opening response	Spontaneously	4
	To speech	3
	To pain	2
	No response	1
Best verbal response	Orientated to time, place and person	5
	Confused	4
	Inappropriate words	3
	Incomprehensible sounds	2
	No response	1
Best motor response	Obeys commands	6
	Moves to localised pain	5
	Flexion withdrawal from pain	4
	Abnormal flexion (decorticate)	3
	Abnormal extension (decerebrate)	2
	No response	1
Total score	Best response	15
	Comatose client	8 or less
	Totally unresponsive	3

Note: The Glasgow Coma Scale for traumatic brain injuries was first introduced in 1974 and is used globally for neurological assessment.

With a trend towards user-friendly medical technology and the introduction of standardised advance skills training programmes, current military medics perform life-saving techniques with decompression needles and chest drains/seals within combat zones; usually before patients are evacuated from the battlefield. Oxygen is administered to casualties with low oxygen saturation, those in shock, and to those suffering from traumatic brain injury (TBI). Oxygen saturation is maintained at over 90% for TBI cases because hypoxia is known to compound this type of trauma. Hypotension is also a feature of TBI and in the early stages of wounding can be very labile. If such patients are unconscious with no palpable peripheral pulse, resuscitation is urgently performed to restore adequate perfusion and a detectable radial pulse. Assessment of consciousness levels are measured by reference to the Glasgow Coma Scale.

There are some caveats in using the Glasgow coma scale in early phases of traumatic brain injury, however, because shock, hypoxia, medications and alcohol can lead to inaccurate scoring.

In addition to treating obvious bleeding and trauma, medics need to be alert to the dangers of hypothermia. Nearly 10% of injured personnel are hypothermic (body temperature below 35°C) on admission to a level-three care facility. This can be due to inclement weather in combat zones, such as the sub-zero winters of Korea (temperatures dropped to -25°C on 29 November 1950), or the bitterly cold waters of the Atlantic Ocean. It can also be the result of massive blood loss. Haemorrhage leads to vasoconstriction which in turn leads to hypothermia. This results in a vicious circle because low body temperature inhibits coagulation proteins, thus increasing the body's tendency to bleed. Preventing hypothermia is difficult in extremely cold, wet environments, although some kits contain pre-packed lightweight blankets, which rapidly heat up once opened. In the absence of such kit, it is important to use whatever extra clothing or blankets are available to keep casualties warm. Medics try, sometimes against seemingly impossible odds, to avoid what is referred to as the 'Lethal Triad of Trauma'. This triad is coagulopathy, metabolic acidosis and hypothermia. Pre-hospital trauma care therefore includes integrated damage control resuscitation, which begins at the point of injury.

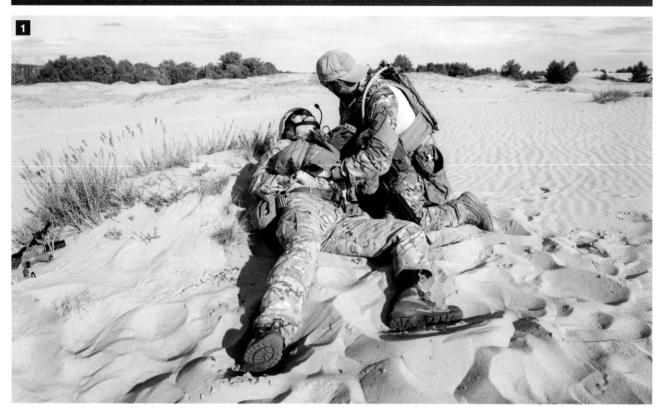

1 Battlefield medicine in the desert. *(Shutterstock)*

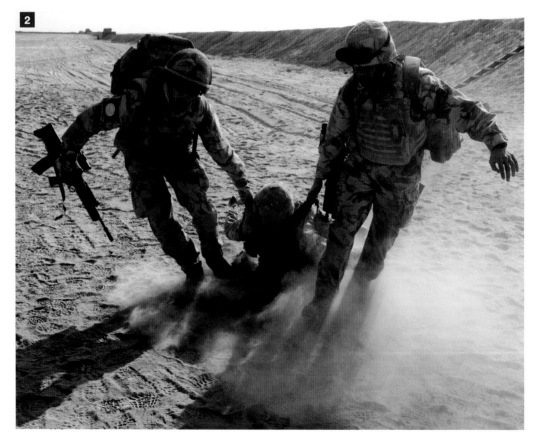

2 British soldiers recover an injured comrade. *(Shutterstock)*

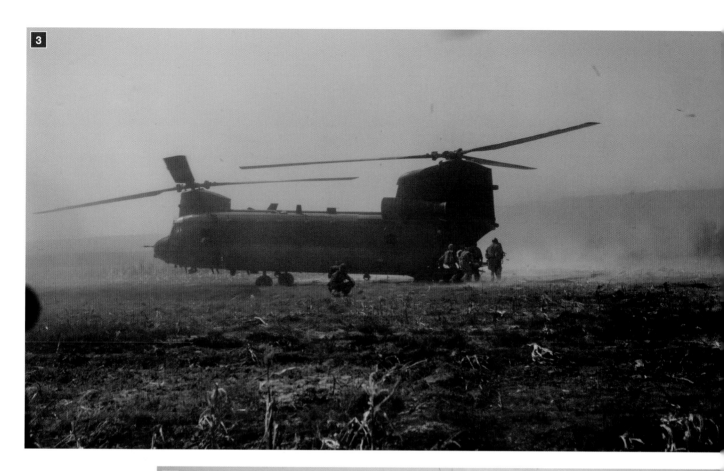

3 The wounded soldier is carried to a waiting Chinook where he is loaded on board for evacuation from Sangin to a hospital at Camp Bastion. *(Alamy)*

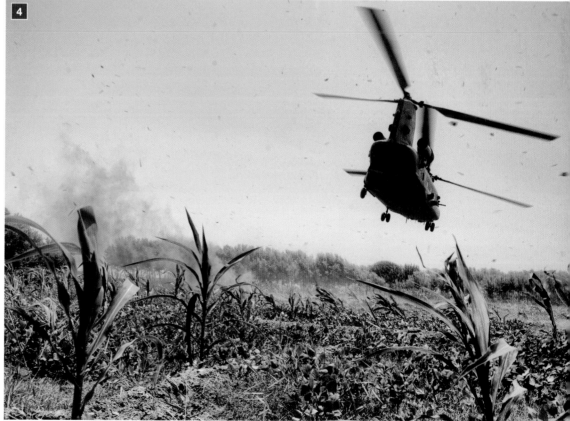

4 With the patient now in the care of the on-board MERT (Medical Emergency Response Team), the Chinook extracts from the combat zone. *(MOD Open Government Licence)*

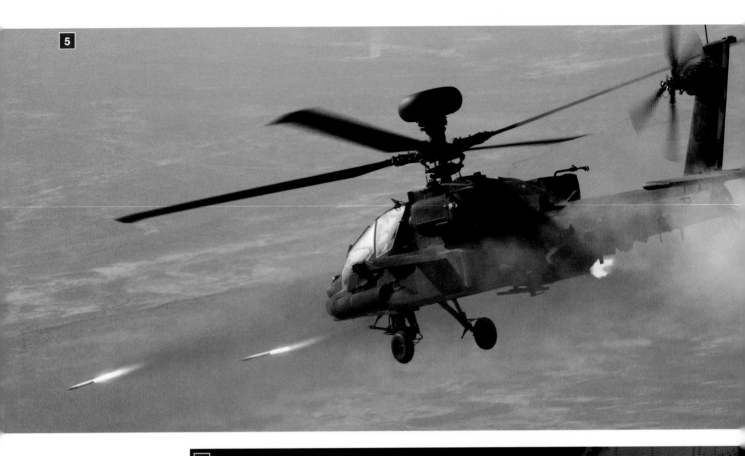

5 Overhead an AH-64 Apache attack helicopter of the Army Air Corps fires rockets at insurgents to cover the Chinook during its extraction. *(MOD Open Government Licence)*

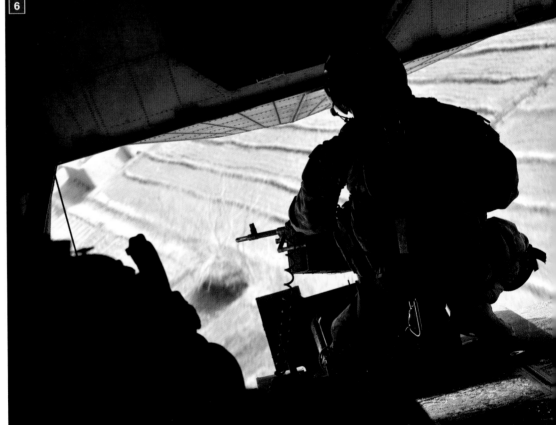

6 A crewman provides suppressing fire out of the Chinook's rear ramp with his 7.62mm GMPG. *(MOD Open Government Licence)*

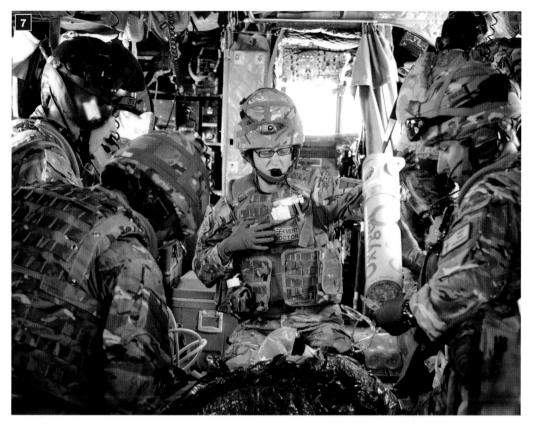

7 On board in-flight, the MERT treats the casualty. *(MOD Open Government Licence)*

8 A crewman voice-marshals the pilots in to land, giving them an audible guide to the manoeuvre. *(MOD Open Government Licence)*

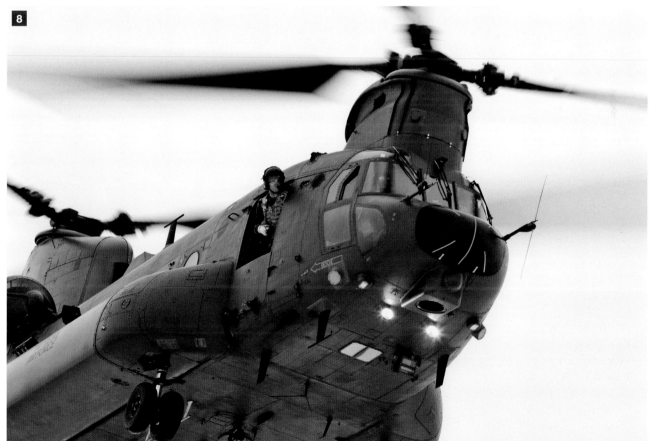

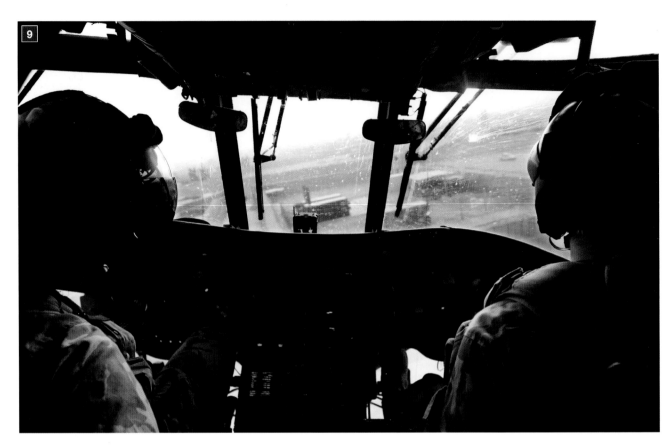

9 The Chinook pilots guide the helicopter gently towards landing. *(MOD Open Government Licence)*

10 Touchdown at Camp Bastion. *(MOD Open Government Licence)*

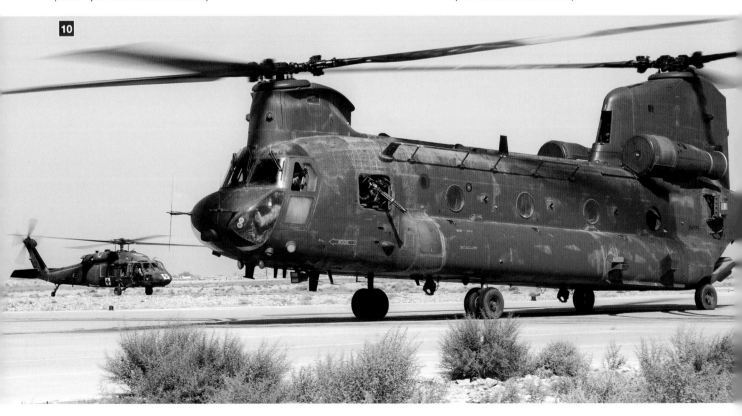

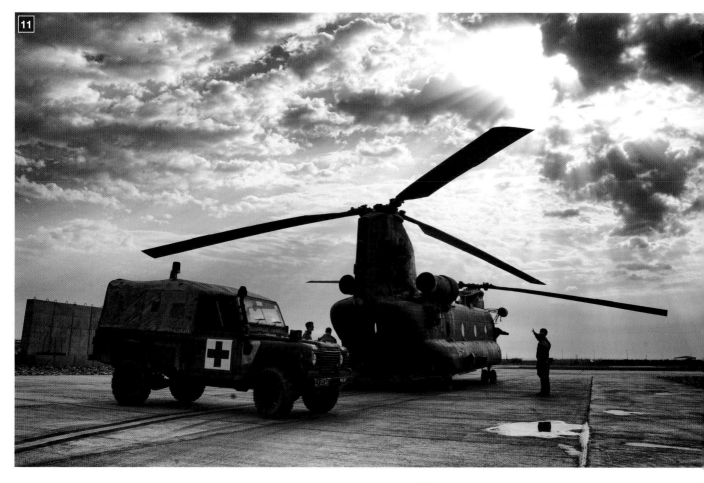

11 A MERT recover the casualty at Bastion ... *(MOD Open Government Licence)*

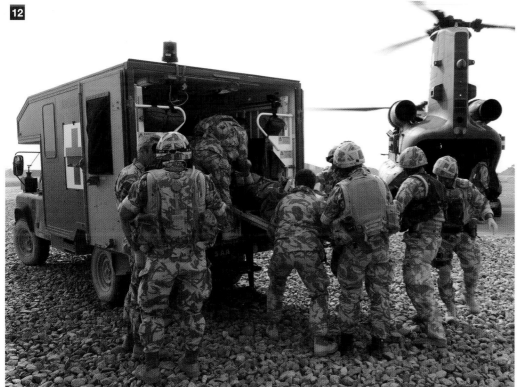

12 ... to a waiting ambulance, which will take him to the Medical Treatment Facility. *(MOD Open Government Licence)*

Delivering this care nonetheless is frequently
fraught with danger and enormous difficulty, as
Charlotte Thompson-Edgar discovered during
one of her medical missions. On 24 December
2007 Squadron Leader nurse Thompson-Edgar
was part of a MERT which was called out
to attend to a marine who had inadvertently
stepped on an enemy landmine in Helmand
Province. The blast blew off both his legs and
his right arm. The team flew from Camp Bastion
in a Boeing Chinook helicopter to where Mark
Ormrod, of 40 Commando, was severely injured.
He had suffered a catastrophic haemorrhage,
yet the team had no blood or plasma to give
him – at this time medical helicopters did not
carry these supplies. She recalled:

*I was gobsmacked – we all were. We'd
never seen anything like it. I mean, where do
you start? We had a reservist doctor with
us who was supposed to lead the treatment
and he just froze – literally for about five
minutes he couldn't move because he was
so overwhelmed. So, me and a paramedic
took a deep breath and got to work on
Mark as the helicopter flew back to Camp
Bastion. We needed to get a fluid line into*
*Mark but the veins in his remaining arm
were flat. Our only option was to perform an
intraosseous infusion, which means drilling
through a patient's bone to deliver fluids. Our
usual landmarks are through the arms and
legs, but because of Mark's injuries, the only
option was to go through a part of his pelvis
called the iliac crest. It is a nerve-racking
procedure because you've got a lot of vital
organs in that area. So that is what me and
the paramedic Corporal Keith Jones did.
He went in one side and I tried the other.
Eventually we got it right.*[5]

Intraosseous infusions are occasionally
administered via the sternum, but this is
precluded in cases of torso trauma. In addition
to providing much-needed fluid resuscitation,
the infusions are also used to give antibiotics
and pain relief; 5mg of morphine is initially given
as a bolus and repeated every ten minutes to
alleviate pain. It is normally given in conjunction
with four-hourly promethazine to avoid nausea.
Since morphine depresses breathing, casualties
need to be carefully monitored and drug
dosage recorded. Tetanus shots are given as a
precautionary measure and essential information

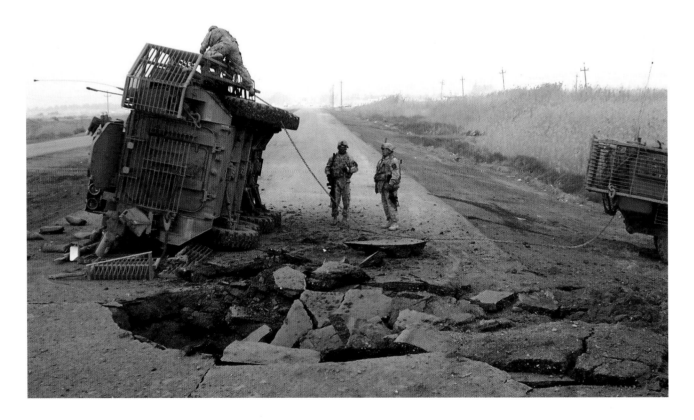

is normally written on the patient's body in pre-hospital trauma situations. Handover in emergency departments follows the ATMIST mnemonic: **a**ge, **t**ime of injury, **m**echanism of injury, **i**njuries seen or suspected, **s**igns and symptoms and **t**reatment given. This triage sieve provides a safe and rapid assessment of multiple casualties into treatment and/or evacuation priorities.[6] Pre-hospital care also entails the splinting of fractures, checking for a peripheral pulse, immobilisation of spinal injuries and stabilisation of head and neck injuries in cases of blunt trauma (*eg* being in a vehicle explosion). Penetrating eye wounds are covered with eye shields and burns covered with dry dressings. If burns are to the face or neck area, then airways may be blocked. Total body surface area of burns is calculated and fluid resuscitation administered.

Occasionally injured personnel will demonstrate signs of mental instability, usually as a result of shock, pain or adverse reactions to drugs. Since such cases pose a significant risk to the casualty and those surrounding him, a medic needs to disarm the combatant quickly to avoid all risks. There are also instances when combat medics sustain horrific injuries. The case of British medic Scott Meenagh of C Company, 2nd Battalion, the Parachute Regiment, is an example: he was seriously wounded by an improvised explosive device (IED) detonation in January 2011. With exceptional grit and determination Scott managed to apply tourniquets to both of his thighs.

Very few casualties can do both legs, no matter how hard they are bleeding; it is just too hard, and they lie back and hope the team medic can manage it. But Scott was the team medic, so he knew there was no one he could wait for – it was him or no one, and no one meant death – so he pulled each tourniquet tight, one after another. Then he checked what he knew by now to be his stumps, but he'd done a good job and the bleeding was under control.[7]

Scott's nightmare was not over. As his brothers in arms attempted to move him on a stretcher to an area suitable for helicopter pick-up, another IED exploded beneath them.

Scott's stretcher crashed to the ground, and someone fell on top of him and screams

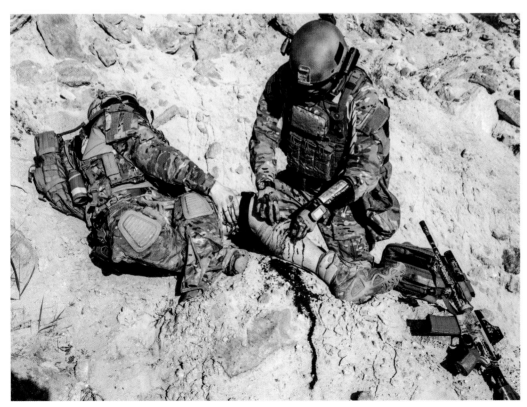

LEFT **A US Ranger provides medical care to a wounded Afghan soldier.** *(Shutterstock)*

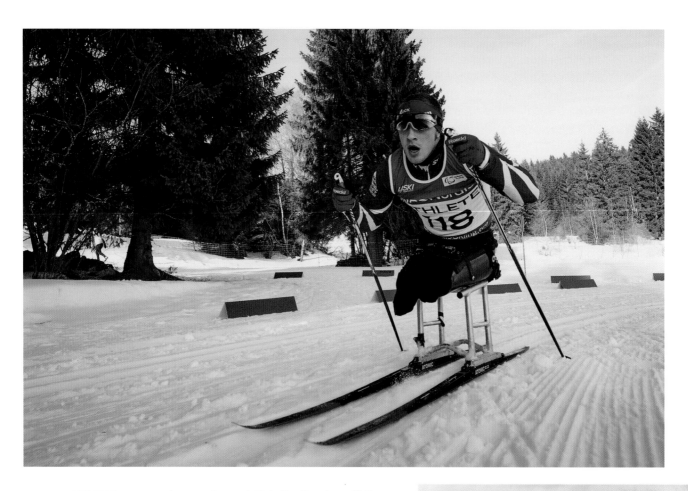

ABOVE Scott Meenagh, who survived serious injuries caused by an IED explosion, races at the IPTC Para Nordic World Championships in Finsterau, Germany, in February 2017. *(Alamy)*

began all round. Only Scott, calm, still the team medic now more than ever, began to call out for each of them to tell him what was happening to them. Four out of five replied. One blinded, one incapacitated, two others peppered with fragments, bleeding. And, worst of all, one silent, the one who lay over Scott, not responsive. Not answering him, except the weight of his body across Scott's a kind of answer in itself.[8]

Scott lost both legs but survived to fight his way back to health. At the 2018 Winter Paralympic Games he became Paralympics GB's first competitor in Nordic Skiing for 20 years and the first ever GB Para Nordic sit skier.

The availability of tourniquets and haemostatic field dressings in soldiers' first-aid kits have significantly improved casualty survival rates. Furthermore, tranexamic acid (TXA), which reduces traumatic bleeding by binding to plasminogen and inhibiting fibrinolytic activity, is highly effective if given within three hours of injury. Protection of blood clots in trauma care is

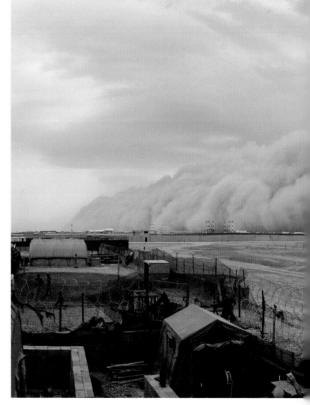

crucial and a reason for permissive hypotension within overall resuscitation. Moreover, there is clear evidence that transfusions of fresh whole blood and blood components improves chances of survival, compared to crystalloid infusions. A study of 59 combatants receiving more than ten units of blood resulted in 86% survival rate and five out of seven soldiers survived after receiving more than 100 units of blood.[9]

Once care under fire and/or tactical field care are complete, the aim is to transfer the wounded to surgical facilities as quickly as possible. This phase is known as tactical evacuation care. During this stage of casualty management medics have greater access to more sophisticated medical equipment and experienced personnel. Joint Allied Doctrine for medical support recommends that injured personnel be taken to a level-two care facility within two hours. Furthermore, according to NATO, extraction time from point of injury to a level-three facility should ideally take a total of seven hours or less. But as the UK Defence Medical Services have stated, it is the first ten minutes of care that is crucial. This is the reason UK medical officers originally introduced the

concept of the platinum ten minutes to save lives, limbs and eyesight. Within this time-frame pathway priorities are assessment, resuscitation and prompt transfer to a facility that can effectively manage the injuries sustained. At care facilities, multidisciplinary trauma teams are led by consultants, and upon arrival, within a two-hour timeline, casualties are rapidly assessed and treated by senior medics. Early triage at the point of injury and tiered hospital alerts are vital, and there is clear evidence that damage-control resuscitation, combined with damage-control surgery synchronously leads to enhanced outcomes.[10] To speed up surgical interventions, medical defence services also established the 'right turn' instruction. This simply refers to the location of operating theatres within the field hospital at Camp Bastion; it means the severely injured are rushed straight into theatre on arrival. Innovations in combat casualty care and training have undoubtedly contributed to lower mortality rates among the wounded. In Afghanistan embedded field medics, the centrality of Camp Bastion and helicopter-borne MERTs have contributed to enhanced outcomes for casualties.[11]

BELOW Extreme climatic conditions frequently added to the challenge of casualty management. Here, a sandstorm envelopes Camp Bastion, Afghanistan, in May 2014. Transported by high winds the sand and dust of the arid Afghan terrain is whipped up, covering everything it crosses. Camp Bastion was handed over to Afghan security forces as part of the planned UK drawdown in Helmand in October 2014. *(MOD Open Government Licence)*

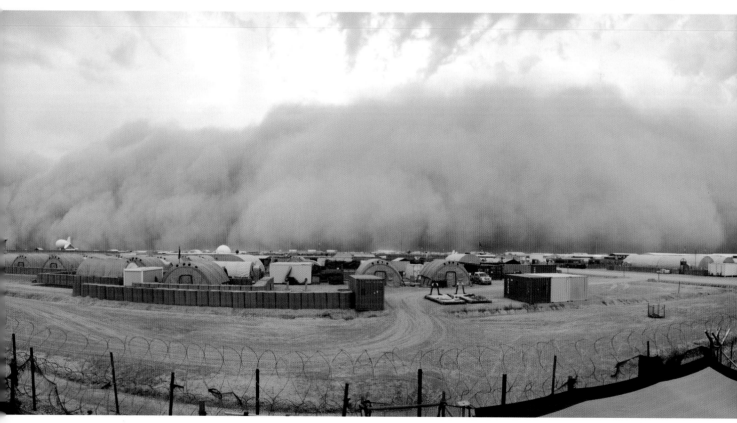

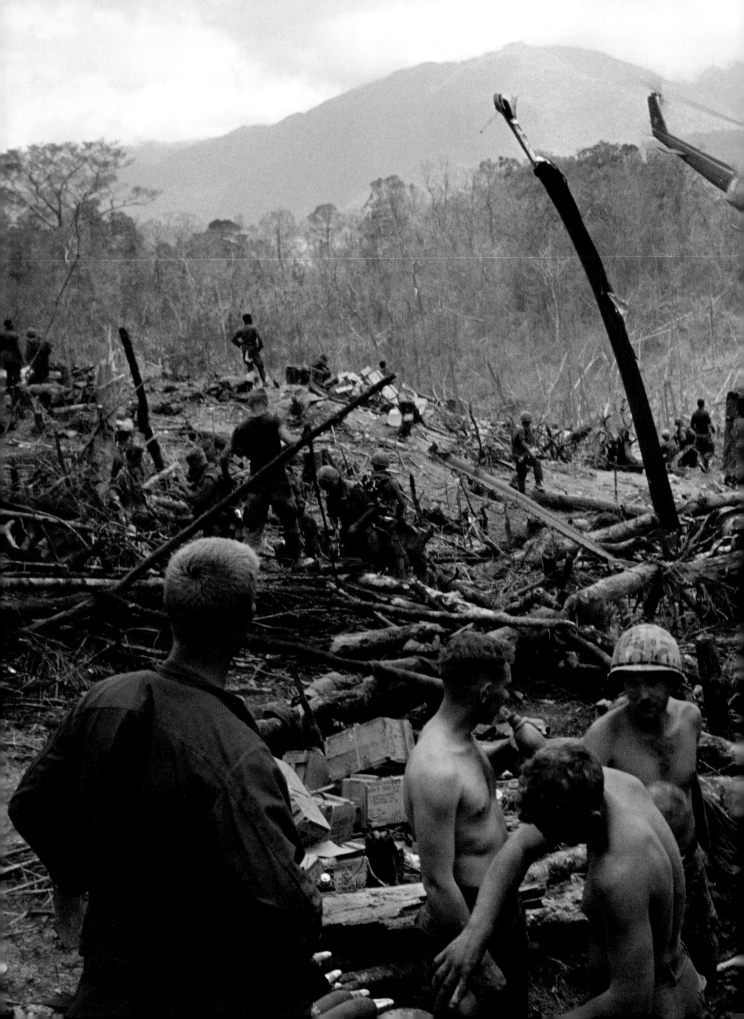

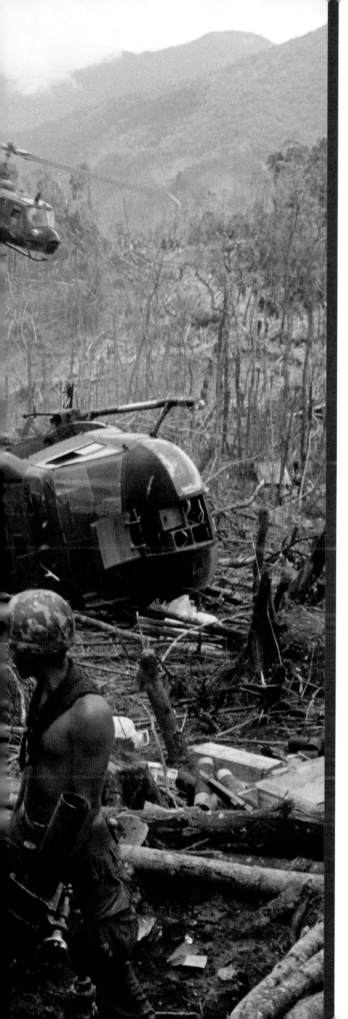

Chapter Three

Evacuation of casualties

Evacuation time frames are guided by tactical, environmental and medical considerations. Aeromedical evacuation is key to reducing the time lag between casualty pick up and arrival at medical care facilities. Furthermore, the concept of taking the emergency room to casualties via Medical Emergency Response Teams (MERTs) has dramatically lowered combat mortality rates.

OPPOSITE Vietnam War: a smoke flare marks the landing spot for a UH-1 Huey helicopter flying in to evacuate US 1st Cavalrymen wounded in the battle for control of the vital A Shau valley on 23 April 1968. *(Getty Images)*

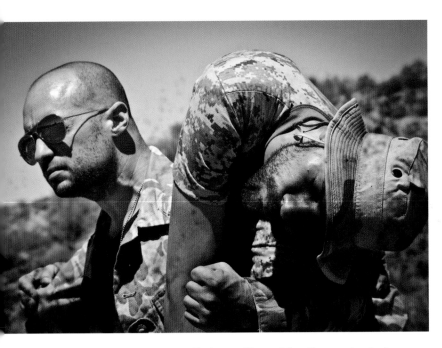

ABOVE **Brothers in arms: a soldier carries his wounded comrade from the battlefront.**
(Getty Images)

Along with providing the very best of first-response combat medicine, safe and speedy casualty evacuation has been key to lowering combatant mortality rates. Lessons taken on board from two world wars – combined with advances in technology – have ensured that time lags between point of injury and surgical interventions were reduced in all subsequent conflicts. The emergence of aeromedical evacuation was the major reason for this time-lag reduction. The first recorded aeromedical evacuation took place on 19 February 1917, when a young airman flying a two-seat BE2c biplane with the Royal Flying Corps (later the Royal Air Force) airlifted a lance corporal with a gunshot wound sustained in a raid on Bir el Hassana in the Sinai Peninsula, to a medical station in El Arish.

There were, however, considerable teething problems with some aspects of air ambulances during the Second World War. Most notably when officials in West Africa ordered several air ambulances, which took months to arrive, and when they did, military personnel discovered that the doors were not wide enough for stretchers to pass through. They were forced, therefore, to rely on the British RAF for the airlift of all their wounded.[1] The United States Army Air Force (USAAF) were also instrumental in ferrying complex medical cases to hospital facilities. One such case arrived in England wearing a blood-soaked turban after having most of his brain exposed in a complete avulsion of the calvaria by a Tiger tank tread; this man, among many others suffering head injuries, was successfully rehabilitated.[2]

It was noted before the Korean War that air evacuation of head injury cases required special treatment and monitoring throughout their journey; they were loaded into helicopters feet first so that they were kept head-upwards in flight. Changes in gravity/turbulence, decreasing oxygen levels at altitude, motion sickness and pressure deviations could potentially cause in-flight problems for patients with TBIs. Low oxygen levels adversely affected respiration and significantly increased the possibility of raised intracranial pressure. The risks of air evacuation, however, were far outweighed by TBIs' needs to have access to life-saving neurosurgery. Furthermore, a British surgeon working in Korea stated, 'I never saw a head injury suffer as a result of air evacuation.'[3]

Neurological patients were not the only cases to require urgent evacuation. Patients suffering with a pneumothorax or other respiratory problems, who frequently needed suction to clear airways and oxygen to improve respiration, also posed a challenge for aircrew. Tracheostomies were performed when necessary before flight and continuous nursing care was provided as required. But unpredictable inclement weather, prompting a need to gain altitude, or situations necessitating quick decompressions were potentially disturbing for patient stability.

Tactical considerations, flying while under fire and poor cabin pressurisation were dangerous conditions for both patients and crew alike. In-flight deaths were uncommon nevertheless, even in instances where total patient collapse occurred. One patient was cleared for flight by his physician even though he suffered severe decerebrate rigidity and had a tube clamped to his chest for draining a pneumothorax. During climb-out, severe respiratory compromise occurred. Fortunately, aboard the aircraft was a physician who could aspirate the pneumothorax and improvise a water seal drainage from intravenous fluid bottles.[4]

Despite the increased use of helicopters in

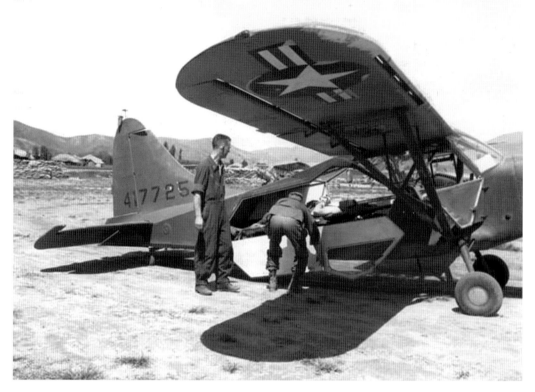

LEFT A seriously wounded American soldier arrives at the US 2nd Infantry Division air strip in the rear area after being flown from the Korean front line in a Stinson L-5B Sentinel observation aircraft, converted to carry one stretcher patient, 30 August 1950. *(amedd.army.mil/korea)*

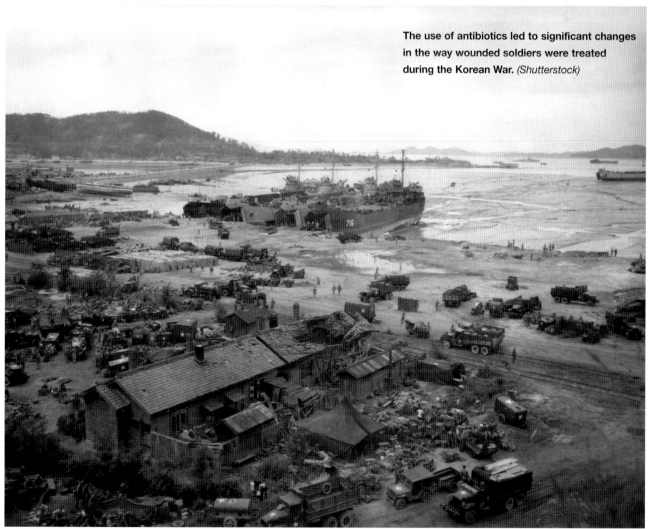

The use of antibiotics led to significant changes in the way wounded soldiers were treated during the Korean War. *(Shutterstock)*

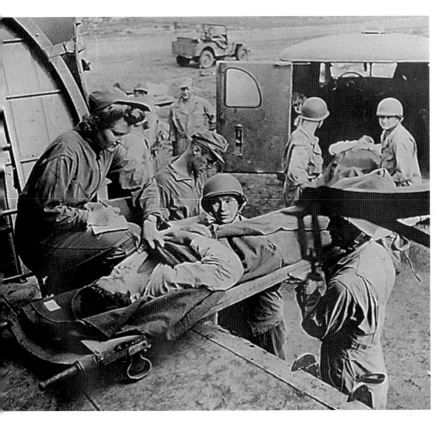

ABOVE Flight nurse Lt Mae Olsen takes the name of a wounded US soldier being placed aboard a C-47 Skytrain for air evacuation from Korea to Guadalcanal during 1953. Due to factors such as noise, vibration and risk of hypoxia, only stable patients were able to be transported at this time.
(US Air Force photo)

Korea, these were only used for the seriously injured. But the introduction of makeshift helicopter platforms flanked on either side of hospital ships enabled helicopter pilots to pick up casualties on the battlefield and get them to a fully functioning operating theatre within half an hour. US naval medical support consisted of three hospital ships and a fixed hospital in Yokosuka, Japan. The latter facility was constantly overcrowded, and patient intake rose from 410 on 31 August 1950 to 1,711 on 10 October 1950. In addition, three medical ships shadowed military activities to provide casualty support. The USS *Consolation* (AH-15) had the capacity to provide medical and surgical care for 802 in-patients and was viewed as a pioneer ship in medical terms. It was the first hospital ship to arrive in Korean waters following its departure from San Francisco in July 1950 and led the way in incorporating female doctors. In addition, the *Consolation* pioneered the use of blood banks as a standard resource, and the introduction of electroencephalographs at sea. In 1951 the vessel became the envy of its counterparts when a helicopter flight deck measuring 60ft in length was installed. This enabled the ship to receive casualties straight from the battlefield.

RIGHT The 15,000-ton USS *Consolation* was the first hospital ship to be fitted with a helicopter landing pad. She had beds for 802 patients and served in the Korean theatre from 1950 to 1954.
(Getty Images)

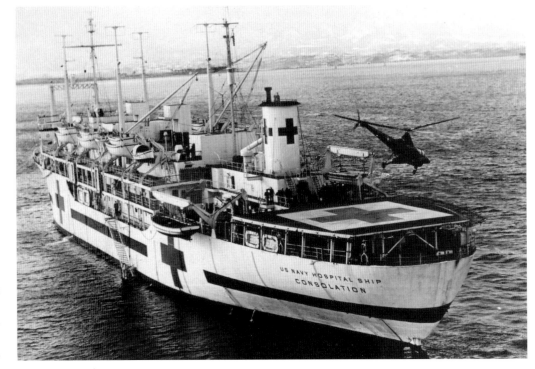

During the first month of tactical operations at Inchon between 25 June and 25 July 1952, 855 patients were admitted to the USS *Repose*. Of this number 705 were received by boat and 150 by helicopter. Most of those admitted from helicopter rescues were critical and receiving blood and oxygen upon arrival. Blood containers were strapped to the sides of helicopters and continuous transfusions given intravenously. Litter handles were equipped with blood bottle racks for ease of patient transfer and aeromedical casualties arriving at hospital ships were rushed into resuscitation/operating rooms in under two minutes. These were located near the middle of the ship because they were less likely to be disturbed by movement in high seas and rough weather. Strategic positioning of hospital ships was crucial to receiving the wounded quickly, and they were deliberately anchored within 30 minutes' flight time of tactical offensives.

With a bed capacity of 750 the USS *Repose* (AH-16) served as a casualty transport vessel and was fitted with a helicopter pad in 1953. The USS *Haven* (AH-12), meanwhile, was able to admit 800 patients and initially had floating helicopter pads attached to either side of her hull. Eventually the *Haven* was also equipped with a fixed helicopter pad on deck.

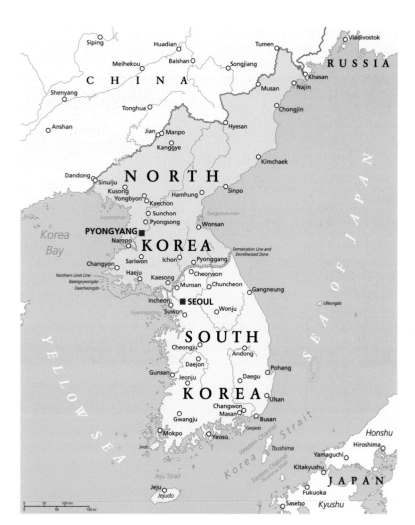

ABOVE North and South Korea.
(Shutterstock)

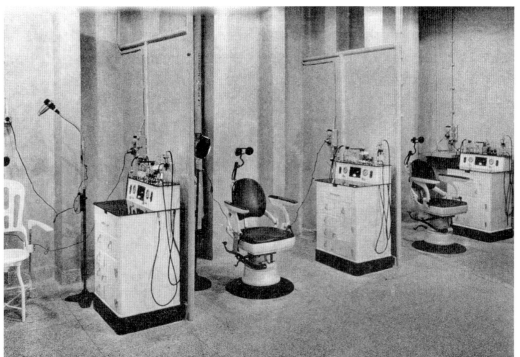

LEFT This is the ear, nose and throat clinic on board the hospital ship USS *Repose*. Hearing problems were common in casualties evacuated from the front line, with perforated ear drums being the most prevalent of conditions.
(US Navy photo)

Korean Conflict	US Naval Medical Support
1950	
25 June North Korean Forces invade South Korea 1 July First US troops arrive in Korea	16 August USS *Consolation* (AH-15) is diverted to Pusan because of infiltration of North Korean communists
	17 August USS *Consolation* is station hospital in Pusan to treat UN casualties
	4 September *Consolation* is diverted to Kobe
	10 September *Consolation* arrives in Yokosuka, Japan
15 September Successful US X Corps on amphibious assault on Inchon UN forces break out of Pusan and move towards 38th Parallel	15 September *Consolation* arrives in Inchon, Korea. USS *Haven* (AH-12) replaces the sunken USS *Benevolence*
18 September US First Marine Division attacks Inchon and Seoul	*Consolation* receives wounded from Inchon and Seoul
	20 September USS *Repose* (AH-16) arrives in Pusan
	2 October *Haven* departs Pearl Harbor for Japan
	18 October *Haven* arrives in Inchon
20 October Pyongyang falls to UN forces	
	25 October *Haven* receives UN casualties, average patient count of 530 patients for a period of six weeks 27 October *Consolation* arrives in Wonsan 4 November 64 patients evacuated from *Consolation* 13 November *Repose* arrives in Inchon 19 November *Haven* patient count is 778. *Repose* leaves Inchon 23 November *Repose* arrives in Chinnampo. *Consolation* travels to Hungnam.
25 November 5th and 7th Marine Regiments reach Yudam-ni 26 November 8th Army is pushed back from Yalu and begins retreating to the south 27 November Chosin Reservoir CCF strike. Chinese lead assaults on leading elements of 5th and 7th Marines 28 November Members from 41 Independent Commando Royal Marines arrive at Koto-ri 29 November Task Force Drysdale moves north to reinforce Hagaru-ri. Column sustains 321 casualties, and 61 Royal Marines are killed in action	
	1 December *Repose* leaves Chinnampo with 752 wounded on board 2 December *Consolation* at Hangnam with 648 patients. *Repose* arrives at Inchon
3 December Pyongyang recaptured by CCF 6 December 5th and 7th Marines attack towards Koto-ri 10 December Forward sections of 5th and 7th Marines reach port at Hangnam and 1st Marine Division suffers 11,731 casualties 24 December 10th Corps US Army evacuate Hangnam and Wonson	

Korean Conflict	US Naval Medical Support
1951	
1–4 January Communists on the offensive reach outskirts of Seoul 4 January US and UN forces evacuate Seoul 5 January Seoul falls to the communist army	*Haven* anchored in Inchon *Repose* anchored in Inchon near gunfire and explosions *Haven* is 12 miles from Inchon
6 January City of Inchon is under fire and abandoned	7 January *Repose* and all UN vessels leave enemy-occupied Inchon port
	8 and 9 January *Haven* and *Repose* arrive in Pusan
	15 January *Consolation* arrives in Pusan 21 January *Repose* leaves Pusan with 301 casualties on board 2 February *Consolation* has 648 casualties
4 February Communist offensive	*Haven* travels to Pusan to aid *Consolation*. Very heavy casualties, with at least 700 received 6 February *Haven* arrives in Pusan, within one day deals with 506 patients 14 February *Haven* travels to Inchon
14 March UN troops retake Seoul	*Repose* leaves Pohang-Dong with 330 casualties
26 April Strong communist offensive inflicts high casualty rates in UN forces	*Haven* in Pusan Heavy, serious casualties, needing urgent surgery and significant medical attention. Staff work 24-hour shifts, and ship is in port for 120 days dealing with overwhelming numbers of wounded. Patients requiring more than 15 days' attention evacuated to Japan
	27 April *Repose* leaves Pusan with 741 casualties. 5 June *Haven*'s patient intake reaches 585.
13 June UN forces retake Pyongyang	
	22 August *Repose* arrives in Pusan 7 October *Repose* leaves Pusan with 140 casualties 9 October *Repose* arrives in Yokosuka to transfer patients to naval hospital because jellyfish have blocked ship's water and sewer lines. High-pressure water is used to unblock the lines and crew are sent on leave 22 October *Repose* returns to Pusan
1952	
	22 January *Repose* leaves Pusan to return to Long Beach 12 February *Repose* arrives at Long Beach for maintenance work and installation of helicopter deck
17 July–4 August Battle for outpost Old Baldy 8 October UN calls indefinite recess 14 October–25 November Battle for Triangle Hill, largest and most costly of the Korean War	
1953	
5 March Joseph Stalin dies 25 March Battle of Pork Chop Hill 27 July Korean War ends. Armistice signed in Panmunjom	

Source: US Navy Bureau of Medicine and Surgery Archives

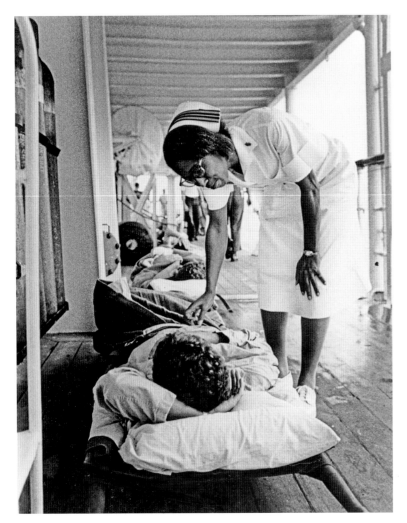

ABOVE A Navy nurse
offers encouragement
to a patient about to
leave ship for further
treatment in the US.
(US Navy photo)

Before the *Repose* was fitted with a helicopter deck in June 1952, the Commanding Officer, Captain E.B. Coyle, improvised loading methods:

> *The* Repose *is equipped with eight litter hoists. Two are located on the after part of the main deck. The remaining six are located on the upper deck. Practically all litter patients have been loaded using the single litter hoist. Litters are then carried into the forward lobby and classified for hospitalisation. At Chinnampo 752 casualties were loaded in forty-eight hours. Litters were loaded using the single hoist on each side of the ship. The lift on the main deck is thirty-seven feet above water. Loading with litter hoists onto the upper deck involves an additional risk; they are located about sixteen feet higher.*[6]

The Commanding Officer of the *Haven*, meanwhile, had created novel helicopter decks by mooring barges to the ship's sides. Without helicopter rescue evacuation, times averaged between four to six hours. It was also clear that some of the wounded would not have survived without helicopter assistance. Sergeant Nicholas Gervase was a machine gunner, injured in an assault near Bunker Hill:

> *We were issued with flak jackets in July 1952, and fortunately I was wearing mine that day. A mortar shell landed right next to me and blew in the right side of my chest. A corpsman held my chest together and kept me alive on Bunker Hill. Who he was is a complete mystery to me; I have no idea what his name was or if he survived this action. I was carried half a mile through a minefield. My stretcher was placed on a rack in a jeep. The road was so rough I could not make this trip. The medical personnel flagged an evac helicopter. They transferred me into the wire basket on the outside of the helicopter. This helicopter had a large plexi-type bubble for the pilot. There was a wire basket each side. I was flown to a field hospital. It was several days before I was taken to a hospital ship. When my stretcher was carried aboard the* Haven *and I saw the nurses in their crisp white uniforms I thought I died and went to heaven.*[7]

Captain Brooks of the *Consolation* recalled that UN troops included a wide variety of service personnel:

> *We had patients from all services and all nationalities. There was a tremendous number of different languages and diets. It wasn't easy. They tried to have interpreters for each nationality. We had Colombians, Turks, Spaniards, Frenchmen and Italians. The British, Scots and Australians were easy. It was always hard for the Turks. When we went from patient to patient, I can remember vividly how we'd have to go from one language to another. Sometimes we'd have to go through four languages before we could speak to the patient. We could see the terror in their eyes. They didn't understand what was going to happen to them. Of course, a lot of them weren't conscious enough to hear anything.*[5]

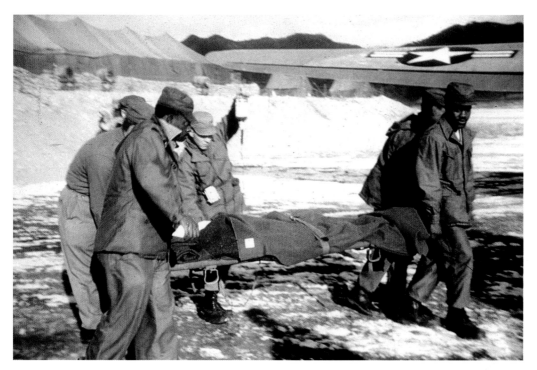

LEFT AND BELOW
US airmen load
American and Allied
casualties on to a US
Air Force Douglas
C-54D Skymaster
transport aircraft at
Taegu Air Base, Korea,
in 1951. *(US Air Force*
photo)

By the 1960s response times for air evacuation were reduced by the introduction of long-range radio equipment. The radio signal 'DUST OFF' (Dedicated, Unhesitating Service to Our Fighting Forces) became the standard military call for air assistance. Once this signal was received it took less than ten minutes for a MEDEVAC to take off to retrieve casualties. Once the wounded were on board, radio contact enabled aircrew to issue updates on their condition while travelling towards hospital facilities. The Bell UH-1 reduced pick-up times in Vietnam, and by 1968 no fewer than 116 medically equipped helicopters were in use. Flying conditions were far from ideal, however, and instrumentation was basic.

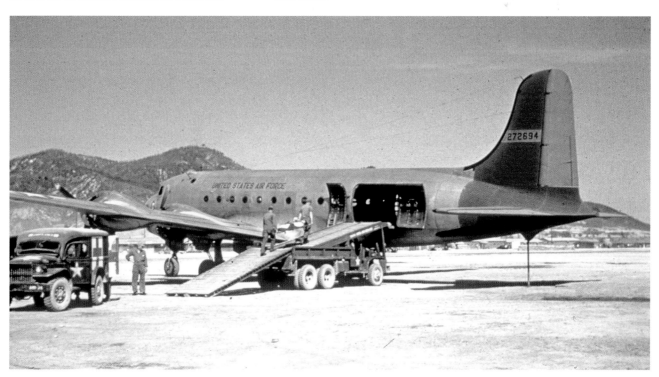

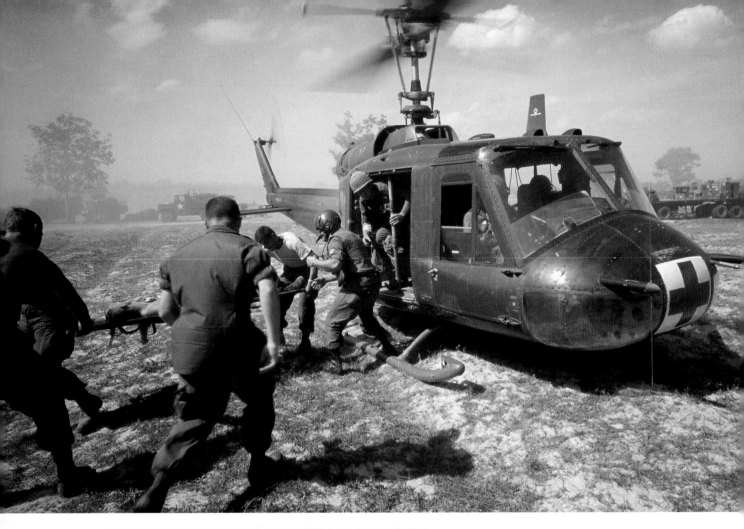

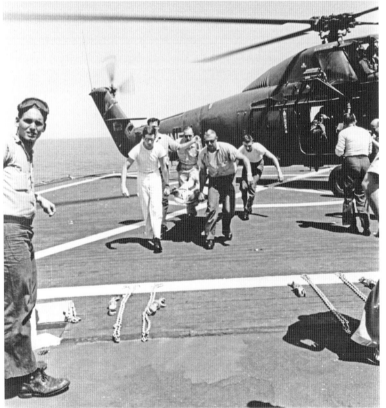

ABOVE An injured serviceman is stretchered off a UH-1 Huey aero-medical evacuation DUST OFF at a medical facility in Vietnam after being airlifted from the battlefield. DUST OFF was the call sign adopted by unarmed US helicopter ambulance units in Vietnam for emergency evacuation of patients from a combat zone. The helicopter crew comprised two pilots, a medic and a crew chief. *(Copyright unknown)*

US Chief Warrant Officer Michael Novosel led the aeromedical evacuation crew DUST OFF 88th and 82nd Medical Detachment, 45th Medical Company, 68th Medical Group. He described the problems encountered when flying in Kien Tuong Province:

LEFT Vietnam: medical assistants aboard USS *Repose* remove a wounded man from a US Marine Corps Sikorsky H-34 rescue helicopter, February 1967. *(US Navy photo)*

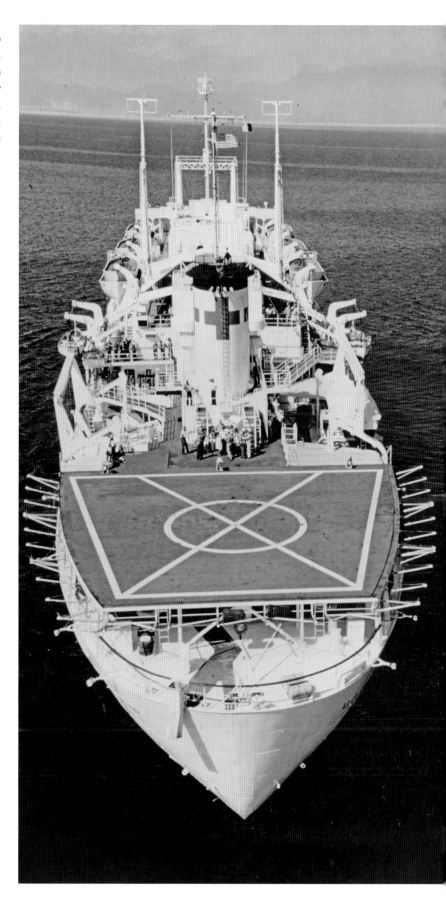

Our people would go out and they would hit thunderstorms and suffer turbulence. Sometimes they would actually punch through to break out into relatively smooth air. Certainly, it was not clear because there was no moon. There was always an overcast and the lighting situation on the ground was not there to help them at all. On a heading they had pre-computed, on a time and distance problem, they had pre-computed and continued to punch on. You can imagine what I am talking about . . . individuals who had to make pick-ups at night to LSTs [landing ship tanks], approximately ten miles off the coast. They did this more than once. They went to the island that was west of Huc Hoa. When you think of the distance involved, when you think of the instrumentation available to the people . . . even if they had had instruments on board the aircraft, they had absolutely no training in VOR [VHF omnidirectional range] or tactical air navigation; we were unable to acquire it.[8]

Novosel transported over 5,500 casualties during a total of 2,543 missions. During the fighting at Kien Tong he flew his UH-1H Huey MEDEVAC helicopter across the combat zone to find casualties. On six occasions severe hostile fire forced him to temporarily fly out of the zone, but he returned to retrieve 15 separate casualty loads. He was wounded during one rescue attempt as he hovered to hold his position while a casualty was hoisted aboard. He also recalled escape incidents:

A Vietnamese command detonated mine overturned an armoured personnel carrier. Miraculously there was a GI pinned down by this, but the ground was soft enough where apparently, he did not suffer any real injury. A crush injury has rather latent effects and we were there waiting for this man to be dug out with shovels, this is how tight the man was pinned down. General Depuy was there. This man, as soon as he was free, got up and started walking, and I remember someone hollering out 'Stay Put'. Someone yelled at him to hold his position, I don't recall who it was, probably the medic because he understood the nature of crush injury, and he rushed up to him with the litter and put him on board.[9]

Attitudes towards casualty evacuation shifted enormously during the Vietnam War. Originally patient transfer was viewed only in terms of getting the wounded to hospitals as soon as possible. In Vietnam a greater emphasis on pre-hospital care and cohesive emergency medical systems led to ideas of continuous resuscitation and the first flying intensive care units. Initially aircraft included a basic range of critical care monitors and skilled nurses. In 1968 the McDonnell Douglas C-9A aircraft was introduced into the conflict zone. Quickly named the 'Cadillac of the Medevac', because of the

medical facilities on board, the C-9A included: folding hydraulic ramps to accommodate more stretcher patients, electrical infrastructures for respirators, cardiac monitors and infusion pumps and in-built oxygen systems. Purpose-built holders in the aircraft's ceiling supported infusion bottles in flight, and innovative interiors lessened the negative impact of high altitudes on wounded patients. Separate areas were earmarked for isolation/infectious patients and for those requiring intensive care nursing. With a bed capacity of 40 patients, the C-9A was able to set a new daily record in 1971 by airlifting 88 casualties to safety – 24 stretcher patients and 64 walking wounded.

Helicopters were still the workhorses of air evacuation, however, although finding suitable landing sites in the field continued to be a problem; as did relaying casualties to ships. During the Falklands Campaign, the RAF Chinook helicopter *Bravo November*, moved wounded combatants from the field hospital at Ajax Bay to the hospital ship *Uganda*. Writing about a helicopter that was affectionately nicknamed 'the shuddering shithouse' by those who flew in her, Dr Rick Jolly asserted:

BELOW The McDonnell Douglas C-9A Nightingale made its debut in 1968, landing at Scott Air Force Base III. Created to be a dedicated air evacuation aircraft, the C-9A was equipped with advanced medical facilities and was capable of faster speeds, which made it a welcome addition to the US Air Force Air Evacuation system. *(PRM Aviation)*

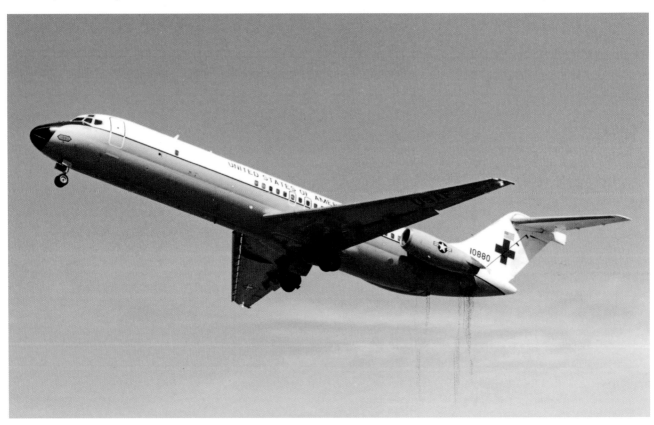

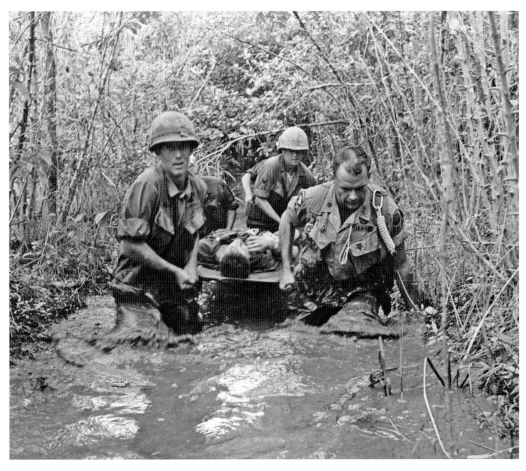

Uganda's flight deck was a bit of a Heath Robinson affair bolted on to the back of the former school's cruise liner. The square landing area was supported by metal struts that projected outwards and upwards from the elegantly curved lines of her stern. The structure could never have received clearance to take something as heavy as a Chinook, but this was war, and the peace time rule book had been lost along with the aircraft's maintenance records and tool kit. The pilot, a lovely man called Dick Langworthy, did a super job of landing athwartships, with only inches between the big helicopter's wheels and the heaving deck edge. Because of the potential weight problem, he maintained some of the lift generated by the huge twin rotors, in a bit of flying skill that could not have been very easy. Both the cockpit and tail ramp were stuck well out over the sea on each side, and the patients had to be carried or led out of the big helicopter via its fuselage side door.[10]

During the 1980s, in preparation for future conflicts, the US military focused on increasing aeromedical proficiency and the number of air-transferable hospitals. Furthermore, holding facilities with a bed capacity of 250 were introduced for casualties awaiting evacuation. The potential for Critical Care Air Transport Teams (CCATT) was also considered. Originally devised by Lieutenant General Dr Paul Carlton, the idea for CCATT was initially rejected by US Air Force and Army chiefs, who believed that air evacuation could not sustain complex critical in-flight care. But involvement in the subsequent Gulf War changed these entrenched attitudes. Large hospitals were constructed near the front line, but the US Army could not depend on the USAF to meet their needs. The C-9A was still operational in the Gulf War, supported by converted cargo planes, but doctors were restricted to ground-level hospitals, making sure that casualties were stable enough for air evacuation. Since medical crews only included USAF nurses and medical technicians, treatment aboard evacuation aircraft was limited.

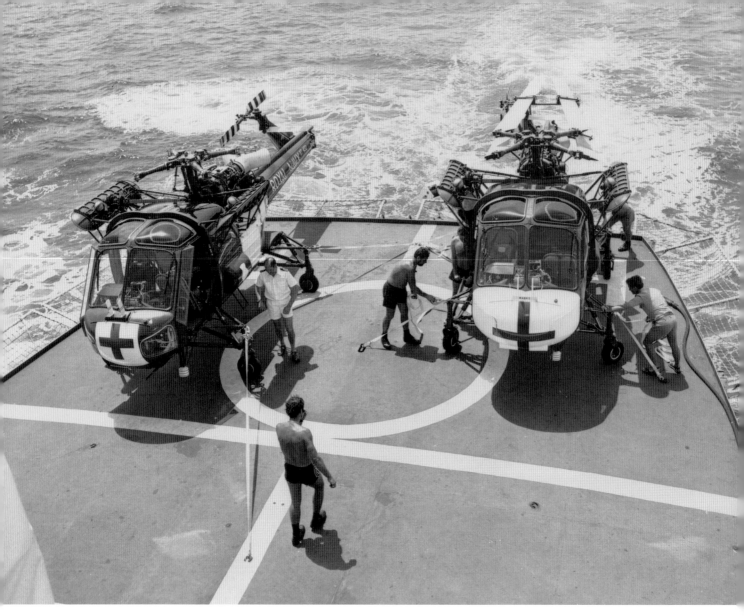

Despite this hindrance, aeromedical teams did successfully evacuate 3,600 casualties a day between August 1990 and March 1991.[11] Nonetheless, strategic thinking surrounding aeromedical evacuations was beginning to shift by 1995. USAF medical services continued to advocate the establishment of smaller hospitals in combat zones, and the introduction of modern transport infrastructures, updated equipment and critical care teams to ferry wounded back to the USA. Army chiefs were finally convinced of this strategic wisdom following an incident involving a young soldier who was electrocuted by overhead wires in Bosnia. He was initially airlifted to Germany and, despite being in a critical and unstable condition, he was then flown back to the US Brooke Army Medical Center. In the aircraft he developed severe septic shock but was successfully resuscitated. In fact, contrary to all expectations, the young soldier arrived back in the USA in a much better medical state than when he left Germany. The case for CCATT was proven. Henceforth intensive care facilities were officially introduced to US aeromedical evacuation systems and CCATT comprised of a critical care doctor, a critical care nurse and a respiratory technician.

With the deployment of troops to Iraq in 2003, co-ordinated information and transmission systems were established to track aeromedical flights and ensure that patient information was quickly relayed to receiving medical facilities. Changing injury patterns affected both the number and severity of casualty evacuations, and critical care teams expanded accordingly. Forward surgical teams, consisting of approximately 20 medical staff,

TOP TEN SPECIALITY CATEGORIES FOR PATIENTS REQUIRING AEROMEDICAL EVACUATION FROM OPERATION IRAQI FREEDOM THEATRE, 2003

Primary medical speciality	Numbers	% of total
Orthopaedics	2,404	21.5
General surgery	1,482	13.3
Psychiatry	769	6.9
Neurosurgery	765	6.8
Internal medicine	695	6.2
Neurology	529	4.7
Pulmonary disease	343	3.1
Ophthalmology	333	3.0
Gynaecology	332	3.0
Otorhinolaryngology	330	3.0

Source: D.R. Harman, et al., 'Aeromedical Evacuations from Operation Iraqi Freedom: A Descriptive Study', *Journal of Military Medicine*, 170 (June 2005). Figures taken from 19 March to late April 2003 – defined as the major combat phase of Operation Iraqi Freedom.

followed fast-moving unit-level engagements, initially reducing the need for large static facilities. But, as the conflict became more protracted, some CSHs evolved into stationary hospitals. US casualties usually stayed in a CSH for three days before being airlifted to level-four medical establishments. Wounded military personnel needing more than a month's treatment were sent back to US Army hospitals. Although lengthy journeys entailed greater risks, as a surgeon reporting from Iraq acknowledged:

Late complications have emerged as a substantial difficulty. Surgeons are seeing startling rates of pulmonary embolism and deep vein thrombosis, for example, perhaps because of the severity of extremity injuries and reliance on long-distance transport in management. Initial data show that five percent of the wounded at Walter Reed [Walter Reed Army Medical Centre, Washington DC] have had a pulmonary embolism, resulting in two deaths. The

BELOW Evacuation in the desert. Aeromedical transfer of casualties could often be delayed in desert situations because of unpredictable and blinding sandstorms. *(Shutterstock)*

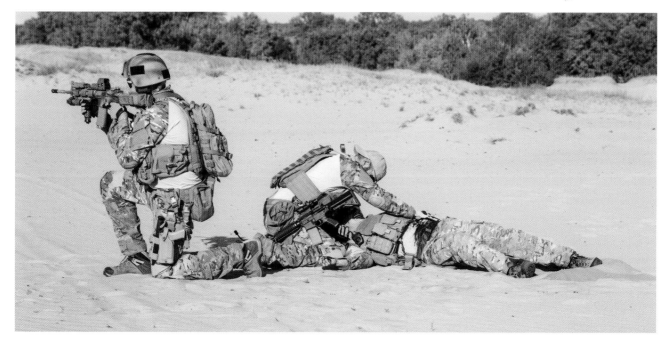

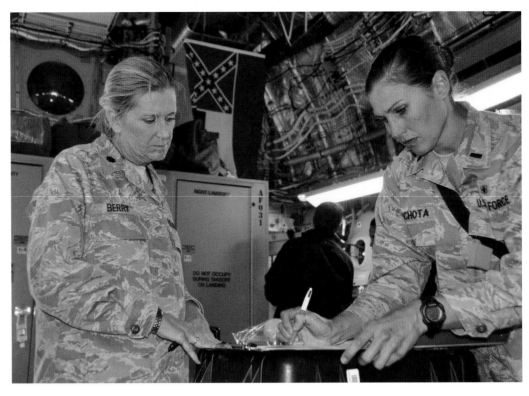

RIGHT Medical technicians assigned to the 86th Aeromedical Squadron at Ramstein Air Force Base (AFB), Germany, review each patient's record and status aboard a Boeing C-17 Globemaster II before it departs during the final leg of a MEDEVAC flight from Ramstein to the United States. *(US Air Force photo)*

BELOW Iraq and its Gulf neighbours. *(Shutterstock)*

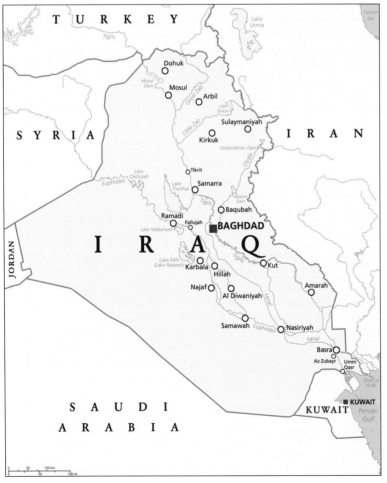

solution is not obvious. Using anti-coagulants in patients with fresh wounds and in need of multiple procedures would seem unwise. On the other hand, there is no facility or expertise in Iraq for the routine replacement of inferior vena cava filters.[12]

Technological advances in aeromedical transfer were a feature of Operation Iraqi Freedom and the conflict in Afghanistan. Aircraft such as the HH-60 Pave Hawk helicopter, C-17 Globemaster III, C-130 Hercules, KC-135 and the A330 Voyager were all instrumental in rescuing casualties, along with the tried and tested Chinook.

Moreover, in terms of aeromedical evacuation, the RAF had substantially more experience than their NATO allies, and were clear leaders in medical innovation. In 2008 the RAF evacuated 800 casualties from Afghanistan. This figure rose to 1,313 in 2009, and dropped back slightly to 1,225 in 2010. When evacuations were conducted under hostile fire, cover was provided by Apache helicopters and ground forces, while RAF MERTs aimed to transport the emergency department to the battlefield wounded. Speaking in 2011, Flight Sergeant

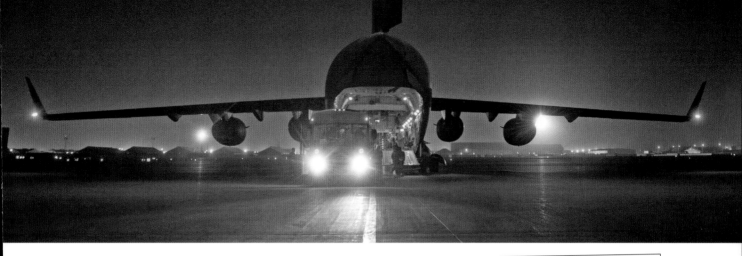

ABOVE Airmen from the 455th Expeditionary Aeromedical Evacuation Squadron and the 455th Expeditionary Medical Group load injured service personnel on to a C-17 Globemaster III aircraft on the flight line at Bagram Airfield, Afghanistan, 8 August 2015. *(US Air Force photo)*

Kevin Swift stated: 'With an anaesthetist, nurse and two paramedics on board and the kit that we've got, it's far superior to what guys had in World War Two and even during the Falklands conflict.'[13]

Request for a MEDEVAC is now called a nine-liner and according to current NATO extraction time-frames, wounded personnel should be able to reach a level-three medical facility within seven hours of sustaining an injury. This time lag is usually much lower, primarily because of the success of MERTs. Furthermore, as Wing Commander Bob Tipping explained:

Where possible we tried to keep the pre-hospital phase as short as possible. Where we have air superiority and things like MERT are deployed, point of injury to arrival at hospital was barely more than an hour, usually much less. MERT

NATO – 9 Line MEDEVAC Request

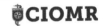

Line 1. Location of the pick-up site.

Line 2. Radio frequency, call sign, and suffix.

Line 3. Number of patients by precedence:

- A – Urgent
- B – Urgent Surgical
- C – Priority
- D – Routine
- E – Convenience

Line 4. Special equipment required:

- A – None
- B – Hoist
- C – Extraction equipment
- D – Ventilator

Line 5. Number of patients:

- A – Litter
- B – Ambulatory

Line 6. Security at pick-up site:

- N – No enemy troops in area
- P – Possible enemy troops in area (approach with caution)
- E – Enemy troops in area (approach with caution)
- X – Enemy troops in area (armed escort required)

* In peacetime - number and types of wounds, injuries, and illnesses

Line 7. Method of marking pick-up site:

- A – Panels
- B – Pyrotechnic signal
- C – Smoke signal
- D – None
- E – Other

Line 8. Patient nationality and status:

- A – Military
- B – Civilian
- C – Non - Military
- D – Non - Civilian
- E – EPW

Line 9. NBC Contamination:

- N – Nuclear
- B – Biological
- C – Chemical

* In peacetime - terrain description of pick-up site

www.ciomr.org   Operational Medicine Committee   v1.5 / 2015

in Afghanistan carried blood and blood products for haemostatic resuscitation during initial evacuation from the field. This was continued in hospital using major haemorrhage protocols and near patient testing with thromboelastography (ROTEM) to guide choice of blood products. Warming of blood and patient is also vital. Damage-control surgery is performed to stop bleeding as quickly as possible. Then definitive surgery is performed later to restore anatomy and function, often back in the UK. Trying to do it all on first visit does the patient no favours. You need to put the plug in and then refill the bath.[14]

Following these interventions casualties were transported back to the UK as soon as possible, both for reasons of patient well-being and to free up bed spaces ready for further casualties. In certain circumstances tactical considerations also influenced the timing of this repatriation process. Repatriation afforded patient access to specialist definitive surgery and contact with family members. Discussion of a patient's medical condition and suitability for aeromedical transfer was conducted by a group of clinicians. These included a doctor with training in aviation medicine and experience, and who had access to other specialists for advice. A medical risk assessment was conducted using available clinical information. If this was insufficient to carry out a risk assessment, then a dialogue was conducted with local physicians, aeromedical liaison officers and the patient, to obtain the required information to ensure the requirements were in place to mitigate any risks posed by aeromedical transfer.[15]

For low-acuity patients the assessment was often completed by the Aeromedical Evacuation Co-ordinating Officer (AECO). A basic proforma was used as a starting point for clinical assessment but was not a definitive decision-making document. Patients requiring intensive care needed more discussion about flight suitability and this was conducted between referral and transfer teams. Wing Commander Tipping, the RAF's Consultant Adviser for pre-hospital care also confirmed that:

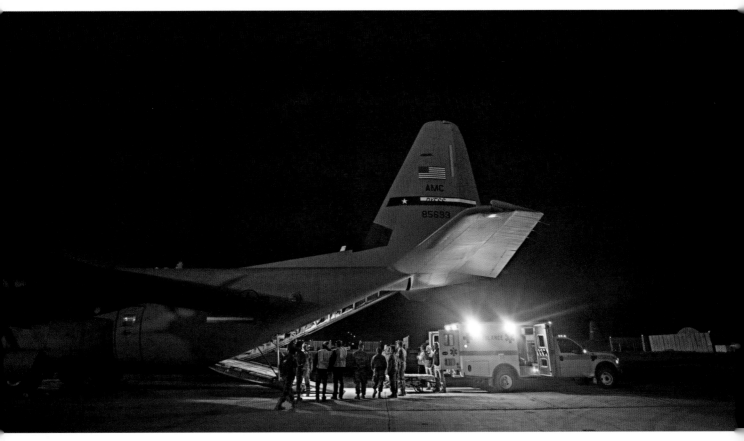

If patients are transported by Critical Care Air Support Teams (CCASTs) they are usually anaesthetised, intubated and ventilated already. On occasions they are awake and have an epidural or other form of pain relief to keep them comfortable. Other considerations surround the surgery and what has already been done. It was not uncommon in the Afghan Campaign for bowels to be stapled closed (after removal of the damaged section) so there were two free ends rather than trying to reconnect them. Obviously, these patients were not able to release any gas in the bowel by 'usual methods'. On ascent to altitude this gas will expand (according to Boyle's law) and can cause pain or perforation. For this reason, the aircraft was usually pressurised to the same altitude that it took off at. Camp Bastion was over 3,000ft altitude. This affects how high the aircraft can fly, and sometimes the route it can take.[16]

In recent years some trauma surgeons have argued the case for permissive hypotension, but this is still a controversial subject:

The jury is still out on how long it is appropriate to continue permissive hypotension before there is inexorable loss of function, especially the kidneys. Even harder if there is a brain injury. Research is ongoing. Keeping the numbers normal is the general mantra for reducing secondary damage.[17]

CCASTs are on call 24 hours a day, all year round. They are not restricted to a certain aircraft and normally consist of six medical professionals: 'a consultant anaesthetist, registrar anaesthetist, two critical care nurses, medical assistant (flight medic) and an equipment technician. This team may be further augmented depending on requirement.'[18]

BELOW A patient is carefully secured prior to an aeromedical evacuation flight aboard a USAF C-17 Globemaster III aircraft from Bagram Airfield to Ramstein on August 2015. The 455th Expeditionary Aeromedical Evacuation Squadron Critical Care Air Transport Team is a three-person, highly specialised medical team consisting of a critical care/emergency medicine physician, a critical care nurse and a respiratory therapist. *(US Air Force photo)*

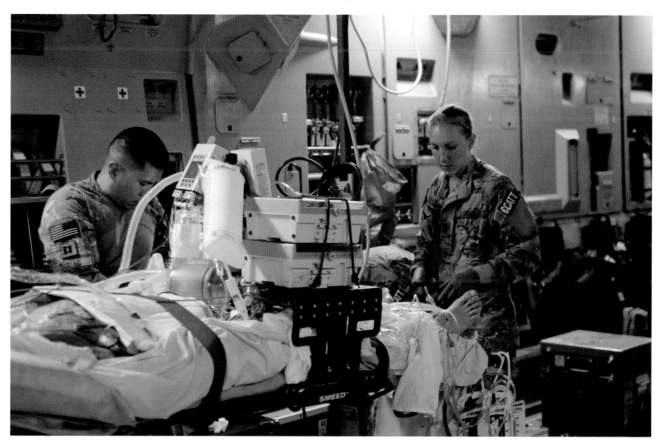

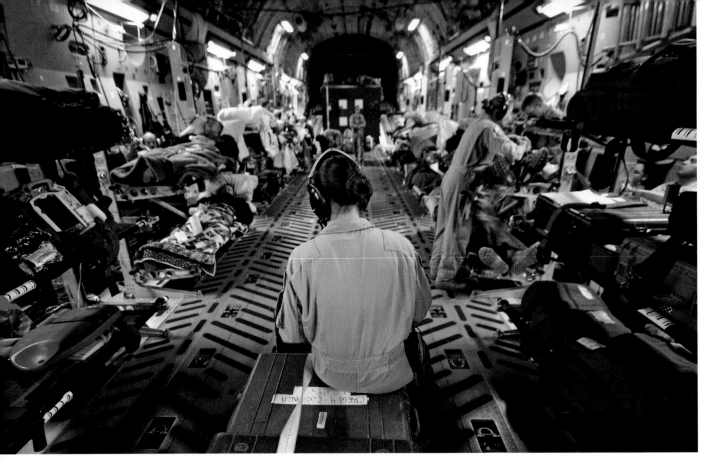

In terms of aviation medicine, the RAF is also at the forefront of research and development. This is aimed at supporting operational capability, human performance, survival and operation effectiveness. Research areas include:

- Increased automation in cockpits.
- Increased use of remotely piloted or autonomous vehicles with associated increase in crewed/uncrewed operations, eg pilots controlling remote aircraft or operating in formations with these platforms.
- Directed energy weapons implications for aircrew and protection systems.
- Unexplained physiological events – working to a better understanding of pathophysiological effects of modern flight patterns and their life-support and protection systems.
- Human health, performance and protection system considerations for hypersonic, stratospheric and suborbital flight.
- Use and limitations of in-flight monitoring, eg wearable technology.
- Information overload – in material to read and remember before flight but also what is presented in flight.
- Shift in live–synthetic training balance.

- Virtual, mixed and augmented reality – implications for training and future (virtual cockpits). Human factors, considerations and medical vision standards to use such systems.
- Protection of musculoskeletal system; prevention of injury as body-mounted or helmet mass increases.
- Use of artificial intelligence, eg to try to predict and diminish reduction in performance or prevent injury.
- Persistent rate of spatial disorientation, research needed to try to reduce this.

Further areas of research focuses on impact protection, high-altitude protection, ejection seat stress/injury modelling, high-G protection for next-generation aircraft, hearing protection for aircrew and maintainers and the effect of flight environment on generally chronic, stable conditions.[19]

Research excellence goes hand in hand with the need to continually update equipment and the RAF recently added the Airbus A400M Atlas aircraft to its aeromedical capability. Able to maintain in-flight cabin altitude at sea level and support innovative technology such as the Air Transportable Isolator (ATI), the Atlas

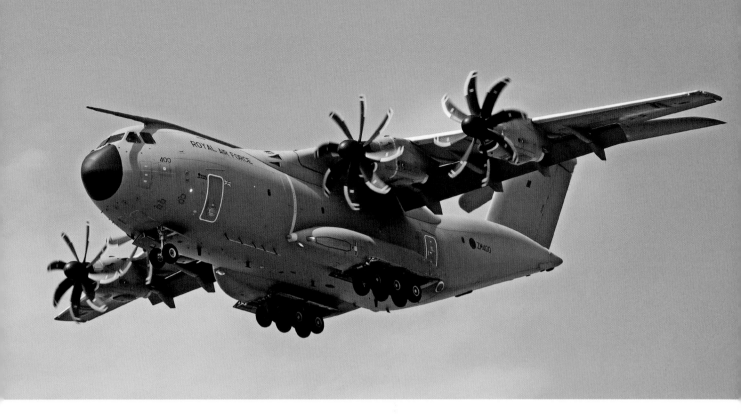

can carry 66 low-dependency patients or 4 high-dependency critical care patients. Being able to operate at sea level provides a safer environment for casualties suffering from lung punctures and TBIs. The ATI, on the other hand, is essentially a safe plastic bubble, which completely isolates patients with infectious diseases, thereby preventing them from infecting others.[20] Medics from the RAF Tactical Medical Wing and the Atlas also took part in the large-scale military exercise Mobility Guardian. This enabled medics to initiate medical evacuations for training purposes, as well as participate in simulated intra-theatre patient transfers. Working alongside US C-17 crews, the objective of the exercise was to train with aeromedical teams from other countries to simulate the evacuation of 300 hospital patients. Exercises such as these

help to determine the medical skills and equipment required in a variety of aeromedical missions. The A400 is symbolic of both the historic role played by the RAF in aeromedical evacuations, and of its future as an exemplary leader in this field.

ABOVE The RAF A400M Atlas C1 can carry 66 low-dependency patients or 4 high-dependency critical care patients. *(Airbus)*

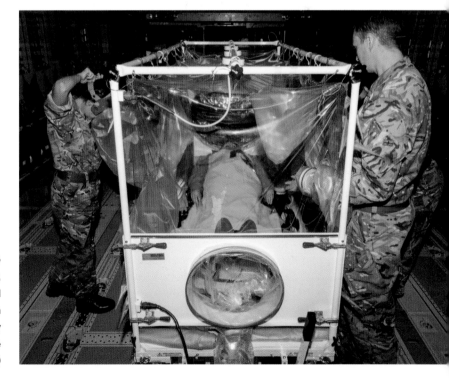

RIGHT In May 2018 the RAF's Atlas programme achieved full aeromedical evacuation capability, enabling the transport of critically ill or injured patients. The A400M Atlas can now act as an airborne intensive care unit as well as safely transporting patients with communicable diseases such as Ebola. *(MOD Crown Copyright)*

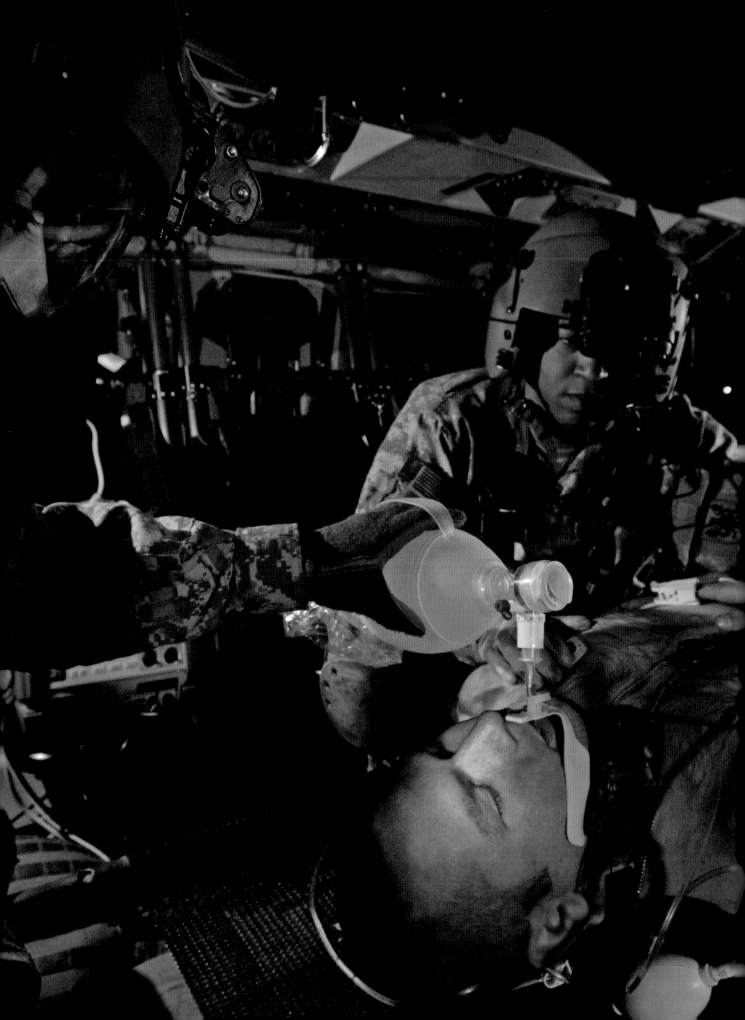

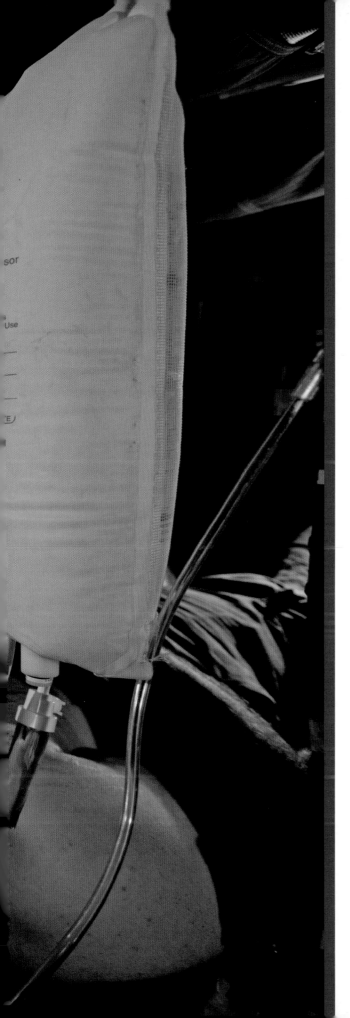

Chapter Four

Anaesthesia

─────(●)─────────────

Defence anaesthetists play a crucial role in tactical casualty management, pain control and the critical care of trauma patients. They are integral to the process of continuous resuscitation, initiated in the Vietnam Conflict, and to the more recently introduced policy of damage control resuscitation.

OPPOSITE A US Army MEDEVAC Crew Chief assists the flight medic by simulating ventilation of a mock patient during training aboard a UH-60L Blackhawk helicopter.

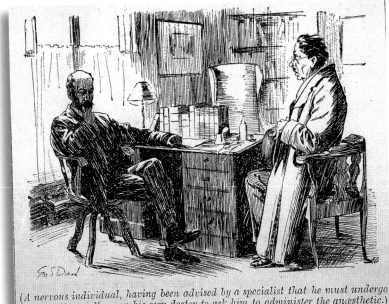

(A nervous individual, having been advised by a specialist that he must undergo an operation, calls upon his own doctor to ask him to administer the anæsthetic.)

The Doctor (a conscientious practitioner). "WELL! I WILL ADMINISTER THE ANÆSTHETIC, BUT—YOU KNOW, I NEVER LIKE DOING IT. THE JURY ARE ALWAYS DOWN ON THE ANÆSTHETIST."

ABOVE *Punch* cartoon – a nervous individual having been advised by a specialist that he must undergo an operation, calls upon his own doctor to administer the anaesthetic.

Within medical circles, anaesthetists have often joked that just as the physiology of the human body maintains a blood/brain barrier, anaesthetists have argued that they provide the brains in the operating theatre while the surgeons deal with the blood. Despite this fact, in the early days of anaesthesia administration, surgical patient deaths, whether civilian or military, were often blamed solely on the anaesthetist.

However, during the 1950s, improvements in anaesthetic equipment, methods of induction, anaesthetic agents and pre-operative drugs drastically reduced the number of deaths caused by patient reactions to anaesthesia. By the 1960s the role of anaesthetists had expanded considerably to include critical care specialists and, like most spheres of medicine, anaesthesia learned valuable lessons from the battlefields.

During the Korean War a lack of trained anaesthetists in forward units severely hampered medical support for troops. This situation was compounded by the fact that neither the training of anaesthetists nor their equipment was standardised. A British gas cylinder coloured green for instance, contained carbon dioxide, whereas a US green gas cylinder contained oxygen. As the US armed forces fought to hold back the communists alongside their allies from the UN, language

problems, differences in power supplies for anaesthetic equipment and variants in medical terminology, all acted to thwart the efforts of doctors serving in forward areas. Even the methods of induction varied from one anaesthetist to another. There was no statistical evidence to indicate the efficacy of certain techniques, drugs or equipment, and consequently individual anaesthetists simply adhered to their own personal preferences.

Nurses were hastily trained in anaesthetics to make up the shortfall in doctors but there were never enough qualified anaesthesia providers in front-line medical units. MASH were effective, but economic constraints often interfered with the availability of drugs and equipment. The British Royal College of Surgeons had established a Faculty of Anaesthetists in 1948 but within the UN Command, levels of competency in anaesthesia varied from one country to another, with some simply receiving on-the-job instruction. Senior US Army medical personnel described the situation as dire; but despite their concerns the Army did not form a three-year residency training programme in anaesthesia until 1954, a year after the Korean War ended.

Some reserve officers insisted on bringing their own anaesthetic equipment with them to Korea; these were mainly machines such as the Beecher device, Foregger or McKesson. This cumbersome equipment was gradually replaced by more compact and easily transportable machinery, such as Boyle's anaesthetic machine.

However, anaesthetic drugs were often shrouded in controversy. For instance, adverse reactions to certain drugs such as sodium thiopental proved fatal on numerous occasions; most notoriously during the treatment of Pearl Harbor casualties during the Second World War. Yet sodium thiopental was a useful and relatively safe induction agent in most cases and in Korea was a common choice for front-line anaesthesia providers. It became a sole agent for light anaesthesia in which operations lasted less than 50 minutes and a frequent add-on to spinal anaesthesia. It was easy to administer and readily available but could not be used for patients suffering from shock, haemorrhage, gas gangrene, impaired oxygen uptake, severe burns or instances where brain surgery was

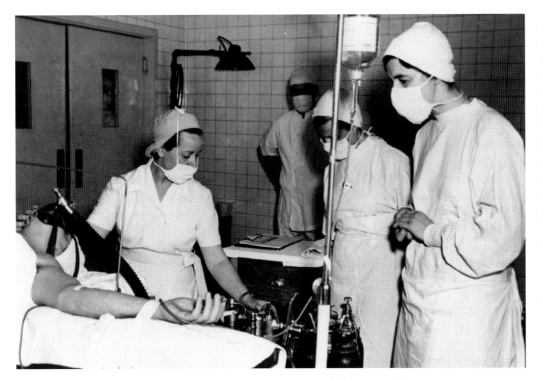

LEFT Captain
Ruth Voelroy, 279th
General Hospital,
Osaka, Japan,
explains how the
Heibrink Anaesthesia
Unit functions to
Norwegian nurses
of Norwegian mobile
surgical units. Nurse
anaesthetists were
introduced during the
First World War but
withdrawn in 1918.
However, the shortage
of male anaesthetists
during the Korean
conflict prompted the
return of female nurse
anaesthetists.
(IWM MH32969)

necessary. Casualties in poor condition simply
could not tolerate barbiturate anaesthesia.
Sodium thiopental, therefore, was more often
reserved for casualties at the rear of evacuation
lines, since those suffering from shock were
more readily found in field hospitals. In addition,
the drug was regularly used as a pre-operative
medication as an alternative to morphine.
The latter was usually given with atropine or
scopolamine, while alternative pre-medications
were normally barbiturate based.

Before the Korean War, chloroform was also
used for induction purposes, but anaesthetists
working in Korea discovered that it depressed
the circulatory system. As a result, chloroform
could not be administered to casualties suffering
from wounds involving their circulation. A
combination of ether, oxygen and nitrous oxide
was the method of induction favoured by most
anaesthetists at this time. Ether did raise blood
sugars quite dramatically and often caused
irritation to the mucous linings of the trachea
and bronchial tubes, but it was also safe and
easily tolerated by most casualties. Rapid
intubation was assisted by muscle relaxants
such as succinylcholine. However, there were
numerous difficulties associated with casualties
receiving induction anaesthesia, particularly if
the casualty was unconscious. In such cases

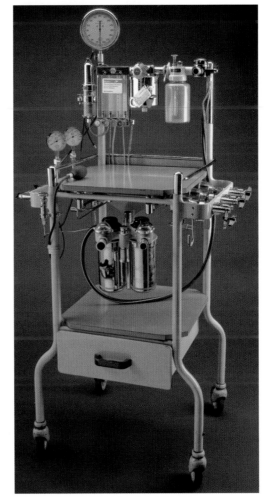

LEFT Boyle-type
anaesthetic machine,
England, 1955–65.
Boyle's law, first
published in 1662,
states that at a
constant temperature
the pressure of a
given gas is inversely
proportional to its
volume. This law
has subsequently
governed all methods
of administering
induction anaesthesia.
(Science Museum)

there was no way of telling if a casualty had eaten prior to sustaining his injuries, which increased the likelihood of tracheal aspiration of stomach contents. Patients with severe burns or muscle injuries frequently reacted to certain drugs, especially succinylcholine, which led to cardiac arrest in susceptible casualties. Compromise or mismanagement of airways also resulted in a number of deaths. Quoting research previously conducted by the British Medical Research Council, Robert Dripps MD, civilian consultant in anaesthesia to the US Army Surgeon General, also emphasised the difference between civilians requiring anaesthesia and those who were injured on the battlefield, noting that:

[. . .] the severely wounded soldier is inordinately susceptible to narcosis regardless of the agent or technique selected. Prior to anaesthesia he presents a picture of apathy and depression suggestive of decreased central nervous system function. He appears to be partially narcotized already. In such a patient small amounts of central nervous depressant drugs evoke a response out of proportion to the size of the dose administered. 'Normal' dosage regimens will cause death sufficiently frequently to drive this point home.

Acknowledging the problems associated with sodium thiopental, Robert Dripps further asserted:

Those men trained primarily in the administration of thiopental soon realised that very small doses of this drug suffice. Profound depression may be produced by 25 to 50mg, if such be the case, it is my opinion that thiopental should be abandoned since nitrous oxide with adequate quantities of oxygen will undoubtedly be all that is necessary [. . .] Beecher has stated that the induction of anaesthesia with ether alone is safe in the seriously wounded. Yet I have produced severe hypotension in battle casualties with this drug in apparently very light planes of anaesthesia. According to recent studies the safety of ether so far as the circulation is concerned lies in its ability

to mobilize epinephrine and norepinephrine from adrenal medulla and sympathetic nerve endings. If this be prevented totally or in part, ether is a potent circulatory depressant. Probably in certain seriously wounded patients such mobilization is reduced.[1]

In the light of experience gained in Korea, several recommendations were made to improve military anaesthesia provision for the future. These included the introduction of a wide variety and increased availability of drugs, standard anaesthesia apparatus and other equipment such as endotracheal tubes, along with standard electrical supplies. Small field anaesthesia cards were also provided for each casualty, which recorded essential personal medical information. By the time US forces became embroiled in the Vietnam War, anaesthetic agents such as halothane, methoxyflurane and diethyl ether had been added to old favourites such as nitrous oxide. There were initial problems with the use of halothane because field anaesthetic apparatus contained in-circuit vaporisers, which permitted different amounts of anaesthetic agent to be determined by pulmonary minute volumes in addition to fixed-dial settings. Therefore, it became almost impossible to gauge with any degree of accuracy the amount of anaesthetic drug inspired by the patient. In these circumstances a casualty with low blood volume and poor cardiac output could easily be overdosed leading to a rapid fall in blood pressure. Nevertheless, as a battlefield anaesthetic, halothane was superior to other agents. Casualties receiving halothane were less likely to vomit after operations compared with those who had received ether induction; and they were more likely to have a good urinary output following the administration of intravenous fluids during operations. Halothane also had the advantage of being non-flammable and post-operative casualties recovered more quickly than with other induction agents. Once the US Army furnished field anaesthetic apparatus with Fluotec MK 1 and MK 2 in 1967, halothane became a popular choice of induction agent, and between 1968 and 1971 it was the most commonly used anaesthetic drug. Moreover, although it was possible

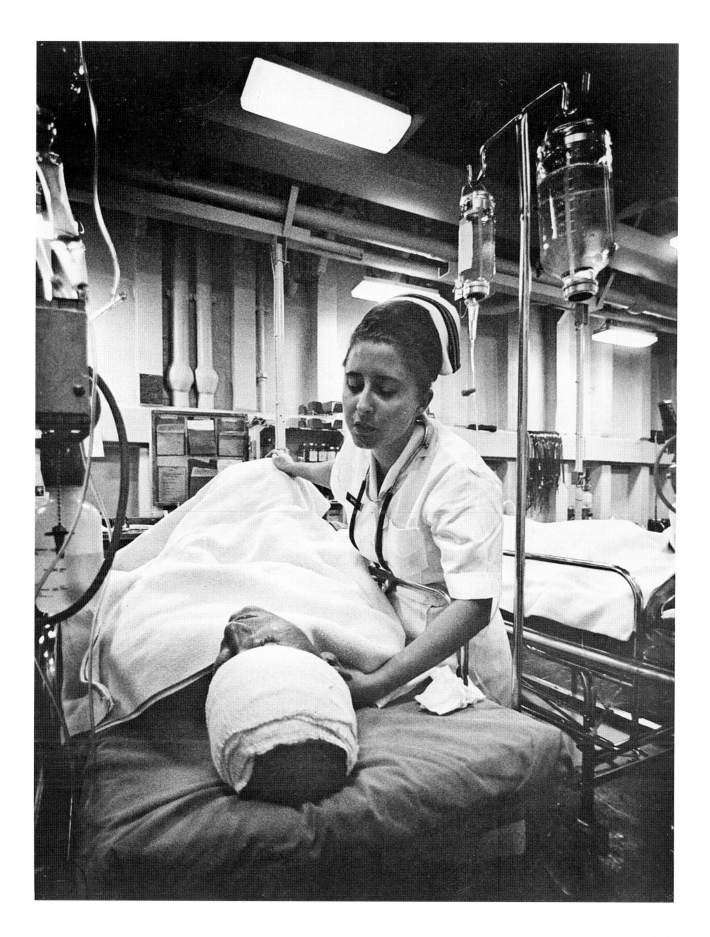

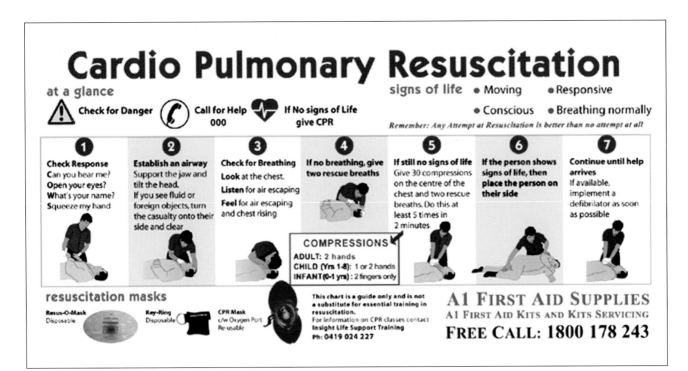

Cardio Pulmonary Resuscitation

at a glance

⚠ **Check for Danger**   📞 **Call for Help** 000   ❤ **If No signs of Life give CPR**

signs of life ● Moving ● Responsive ● Conscious ● Breathing normally

Remember: Any Attempt at Resuscitation is better than no attempt at all

1 Check Response
Can you hear me?
Open your eyes?
What's your name?
Squeeze my hand

2 Establish an airway
Support the jaw and tilt the head.
If you see fluid or foreign objects, turn the casualty onto their side and clear

3 Check for Breathing
Look at the chest.
Listen for air escaping
Feel for air escaping and chest rising

4 If no breathing, give two rescue breaths

COMPRESSIONS
ADULT: 2 hands
CHILD (Yrs 1-8): 1 or 2 hands
INFANT (0-1 yrs): 2 fingers only

5 If still no signs of life
Give 30 compressions on the centre of the chest and two rescue breaths. Do this at least 5 times in 2 minutes

6 If the person shows signs of life, then place the person on their side

7 Continue until help arrives
If available, implement a defibrilator as soon as possible

resuscitation masks

Resus-O-Mask
Disposable

Key-Ring
Disposable

CPR Mask
c/w Oxygen Port
Re-usable

This chart is a guide only and is not a substitute for essential training in resuscitation.
For information on CPR classes contact
Insight Life Support Training
Ph: 0419 024 227

A1 FIRST AID SUPPLIES
A1 FIRST AID KITS AND KITS SERVICING
FREE CALL: 1800 178 243

ABOVE

Cardiopulmonary resuscitation diagram.

(US Air Force photo)

for anaesthetists to administer anaesthesia using a mask, by this stage in Vietnam over three-quarters of casualties received general anaesthesia via endotracheal tubes.

Through military residency training programmes, the US Army produced and deployed board certificate level anaesthetists to forward static hospitals in Vietnam. Following an escalation of the war in 1965, the number of anaesthetists rose dramatically, peaking at 95 at the height of the conflict. Many of these were nurse anaesthetists, recruited by the Army and educated to masters' degree standard. Yet training programmes still varied considerably, and some anaesthetists were sent to Vietnam having received only 14 weeks' training. Thus, there was considerable rivalry between experienced nurse anaesthetists and those who had received minimal on-the-job instruction. Anaesthesia providers travelled between large military hospitals within combat zones depending on the number of casualties and the severity of their injuries. Invariably casualties suffered from deep multiple wounds caused by high-velocity missiles and mines. Amid growing scenes of appalling devastation, the role of the anaesthetist expanded rapidly and medical experiences in the Vietnam War became a turning point in terms of battlefield medicine.

The innovative policy of continuous

resuscitation was first introduced in Vietnam and produced astonishing results. John Jenicek, consultant anaesthesiologist to the US Army Surgeon General, ushering in this new approach explained:

It became the mission of anaesthesia teams to support the circulating volume, the oxygen demand, and the anaesthetic needs of the patient, as well as to treat and correct all abnormal physiological and pharmacological responses of the casualty; all the while providing as near optimal surgical conditions as possible for the other equally busy surgical teams. It is this new concept of resuscitation–anaesthesia–surgery, organised and functioning as a unit (and combined with speedy evacuation), which produced the highest survival rate in any conflict so far.[2]

Military hospital mortality rates were reduced from the 4.5% Second World War figure, down to 2.2%. Ground combat medics gave casualties mouth-to-mouth resuscitation, sometimes performing emergency tracheostomies to keep their airways open, treated them for shock, stemmed blood loss and often inserted lines to administer intravenous fluids. These casualties were then picked up by helicopters with evacuation medics on board. The process of resuscitation continued uninterrupted en route to hospitals. Patients who responded well to resuscitation were quickly ushered into operating rooms for immediate surgery, while those who needed surgical intervention to aid resuscitation were given light anaesthesia. There was a plentiful supply of whole blood and dextran, along with fluids to correct electrolyte imbalance. More importantly, a greater proportion of the critically wounded reached hospital than in any previous conflict. Nearly 90% of those casualties who received hospital care in Vietnam were able to return to duty.

Along with the introduction of new resuscitation protocols, anaesthetic equipment continued to evolve. Whereas the Ohio apparatus was the machine of choice in Vietnam, newer Tri-Service draw-over systems, which used ambient air as the chief carrier gas, became increasingly popular, particularly during the Falklands Campaign.

Designed by the British specifically for military field use, featuring a vaporiser, an additional oxygen regulator, a ventilator and self-inflating bag, the Tri-Service apparatus was portable and versatile. Reporting on medical lessons gained during the Falklands, senior surgeon P.S. London noted:

At a higher technical level it was striking to see what could be done, and how quickly, to adapt unsuitable accommodation to medical and surgical needs – for example, wardroom to ward and disused refrigeration plant to operating theatre.

In these days of technical elaboration and conspicuous consumption it is chastening

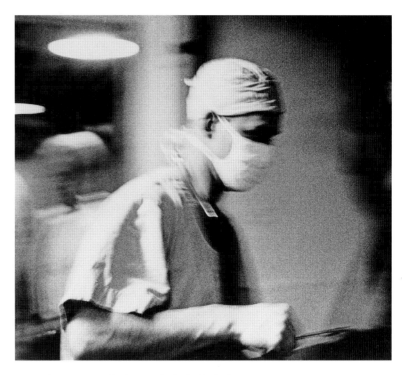

and necessary, to be reminded of what can be achieved by knowledgeable cutting of corners, which can perhaps be more acceptably described as concentrating on essentials when dealing with fit young men. Anaesthesia requires few drugs and little apparatus but, because the anaesthetist may have to use one hand to ventilate his patient and the other to aid intravenous infusion, an oscillometer is preferable to the usual cuff and gauge for measuring blood pressure; the apparatus based upon the Oxford miniature vaporiser and adapted by the medical services of the Armed Forces proved its value. Halothane and trilene were used a great deal for primary operations, regional and spinal analgesia very little.[3]

ABOVE A surgeon hastens to the operating room as wounded marines arrive aboard USS *Repose* while the ship steams off the coast of Vietnam, a few miles south of the 17th Parallel, October 1967.
(US Navy photo)

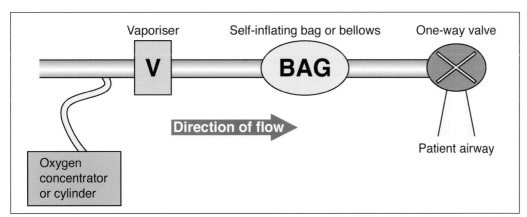

LEFT Diagram of Tri-Service draw-over machine.

Some patients, however, experienced unusual reactions to anaesthetics as senior medical officer Rick Jolly recalled:

Two SAS men had been flown in with gunshot wounds that were quite obviously more than twenty-four hours old. We knew better than to ask them about the circumstances of their injuries, and instead simply operated on them. The anaesthetist, Malcolm Jowitt, used Ketamine, an injectable and steroid-based anaesthetic that has some occasional and highly interesting side effects. One of the SAS men, a big ex-Sapper, came round from his op and started singing bawdy rugby songs, quite tunefully, at the top of his voice![4]

Subsequently, following flawless anaesthesia administration in the Falklands, various configurations of Tri-Service units became the mainstay for UK defence medical services. Easy to assemble and simple to use, they were essential for providing anaesthesia in tactical combat scenarios, particularly air assaults, and for use in remote territories. Future use of Tri-Service apparatus, however, may primarily be dependent on new drugs and techniques. Desflurane and Xenon, for instance, signal a departure from traditional inhaled anaesthetics such as the broadly used isoflurane.

The former has a lower solubility in blood and tissues. This imparts greater control to maintenance of anaesthesia and a more rapid elimination and recovery from anaesthesia. Xenon is more potent than nitrous oxide but not recommended for neuro-anaesthesia because it appears to increase cerebral blood flow.[5]

Transition towards new equipment may also be hastened because existing Tri-Service machinery lacks a CE mark. This means that it lacks European approval and cannot be used within the UK National Health Service (NHS). Since UK anaesthetists invariably gain most of their clinical experience within the NHS, a lack of familiarity with Tri-Service apparatus requires them to undertake additional training before deployment.

Indeed, pre-deployment high-fidelity simulation training was introduced specifically

COMPONENTS OF TRI-SERVICE APPARATUS AS USED IN THE FALKLANDS CAMPAIGN

Medical gas	
Oxygen 0.3m^3 cylinder	1 contains 340 litres

Equipment	
Airways, Guedel, sizes 1, 2, 3, 4	1 of each size
Connectors, endotracheal, 15mm	1 set
Regulator, oxygen	(Houtonox, Penlon 1)
Resuscitator, Laerdal, RFII	(Vickers Medical) complete with adult mask, child mask and extension tube (0.75m). (Cagemount taper connections) extension tube (0.15m) (Cagemount taper connections) plus oxygen adaptor.
Spanner, gas cylinder (Penlon)	1
1-piece connector (Sanders) with gas inlet	1
Cagemount taper connections	Penlon
Tubing, 30mm Lumen	3m
Vaporiser, Tri-Service (Penlon)	2
Instruction and servicing handbooks (Penlon)	1 of each
Yoke adapter, bullnose to oxygen pin index	1
Yoke adapter, US to oxygen pin index	1
Yoke adapter, DIN477 to oxygen pin index	1
Additional items packed in 'Lacon' alloy container sufficient for 10 cases	

Drugs	
Adrenaline injection 1%	1ml ampoules, 10
Alcuronium chloride injection	10mg ampoules, 10
Atropine sulphate	600mcg ampoules, 30
Calcium gluconate injection 10%	10ml ampoules, 10
Diazepam injection	10mg ampoules, 10
Halothane	250ml bottle, 1
Hydrocortisone sodium succinate	100mg vials, 2
Ketamine 50mg per ml	10ml vials, 2
Lubricating jelly	82g, 1
Naloxone hydrochloride injection	0.4mg ampoules, 10
Neostigmine injection	2.5mg ampoules, 20
Papaveretum injection	20mg ampoules, 20
Perphenazine injection	5mg ampoules, 5
Pethidine injection	100mg ampoules, 20
Suxamethonine bromide powder	67mg ampoules, 20
Thiopentone sodium injection	2.5g multidose, 20
Trichloroethylene	500ml bottle
Tubercuranine injection	15mg ampoules, 25
Water for injection	100ml bottles, 3

Dressings	
Adhesive plaster, zinc oxide	25cm × 5m roll, 2
Gauze pads, spirit impregnated	100
Gauze pads, green, 12-ply	10cm × 10cm, 100

Equipment	
Brush, endotracheal	1
Bulb laryngoscope	2
Connecters, endotracheal 15mm	1 set
Forceps, Magill	1
Forceps, Dunhill 130mm	2
Gag, Ferguson	1
Introducer, malleable	1
Laryngoscope, Macintosh	2
Needles, hypodermic 23 & 21 SWG	40
Scissors, blunt point 130mm	1
Sphygmomanometer, aneroid	1
Stethoscope	1
Syringes, hypodermic, 2ml, 5ml & 20ml	30
Tubes, endotracheal cuffed, 7, 8, 9, 9.5mm	1 of each
Tubes, endotracheal non-cuffed, 3, 4, 5, 6, 8mm	1 of each
Spanner gas cylinder Penlon	1
Bodok seal	2
O-ring for bull-nose cylinder adapter	1
Battery, dry no. 9. u ll	4

Note: Transfusion fluids and equipment, plus foot-operated suction machine is also carried in addition to Tri-Service apparatus

Source: Brigadier I. Houghton, 'Draw-Over Anaesthesia Apparatus', 55fst-ramc.org.uk

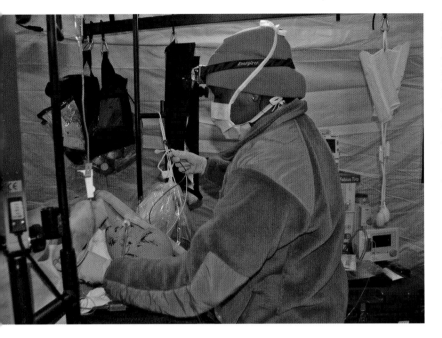

to prepare anaesthetists for severe battlefield trauma. With a special focus on dealing with common blast and ballistic injuries, simulation provides realistic situation-driven events designed to improve decision making, develop and test medical knowledge, gain familiarity with specific deployment areas and practise complex technical skills. Multidisciplinary educational courses were also established throughout the

NATO alliance, to improve overall effectiveness in the field. Furthermore, whereas the intubation process for anaesthesia could prove difficult in some trauma victims, modern equipment has largely resolved this problem. As Wing Commander Bob Tipping asserts: 'Intubation is harder if you can't extend the neck, but ventilation of someone with a cervical spine injury is no different to anyone else. We have Airtraq to help if needed.'[6]

During both Gulf Wars and in Afghanistan, specialist static anaesthetic machines were installed in forward CSHs, along with innovative, intensive care ventilators. Furthermore, with the introduction of damage-control resuscitation, US Army medical services also achieved considerable success in using total intravenous anaesthesia (TIVA) combined with analgesia. Propofol was used as the sedative while pain relief was provided by remifentanil. Patients receiving TIVA exhibited less post-operative confusion and nausea, but it was impossible to accurately measure and control the depth of anaesthesia. Nevertheless, closed-loop, possibly automated, TIVA is currently being hailed by the USA as the battlefield anaesthetic of the future. Research is ongoing and funded by US Congress.[7]

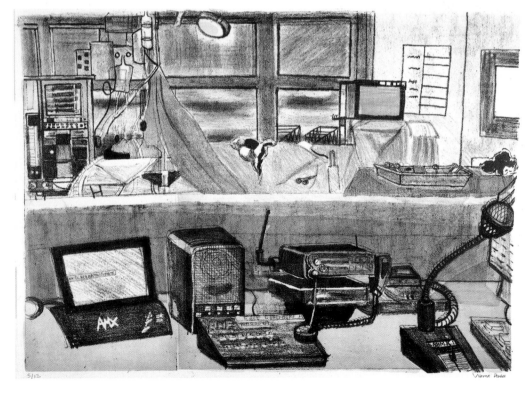

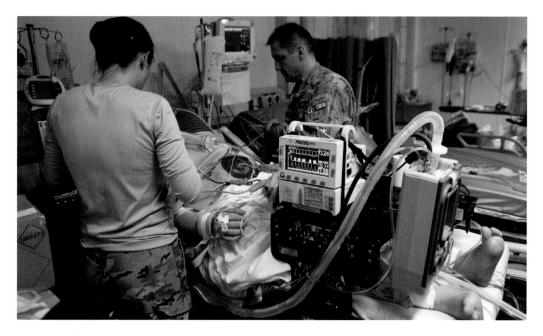

LEFT Clinicians from the 455th Expeditionary Aeromedical Evacuation Squadron Critical Care Air Transport Team (CCATT) connect a patient to CCATT medical equipment at Bagram Airfield, Afghanistan, on 21 March 2013. A CCATT crew consists of a physician, intensive care nurse and a respiratory therapist, making it possible to move severely injured or gravely ill service personnel by air. *(US Air Force photo)*

HIGH-ALTITUDE ANAESTHESIA

Even modest altitude has an impact on available PiO2 (inspired oxygen) and as a consequence a corresponding impact on oxygen delivery. During initial phases of the conflict in Afghanistan, military teams were likely to be exposed to high altitudes (HA); especially if they needed to deploy to or treat casualties at high altitude, including those in transit by air.

Artificial HA environment can be generated by creating a lower pressure, thus lowering FiO2 (hypobaric hypoxia, or HH). This is a highly specialised technique requiring complex chambers and skilled operators. Investigators and subjects are exposed to the same low pressure, giving rise to a risk of decompression illness (DCI) and potential long-term health issues, which mandates tight controls on the fitness of subjects and duration of exposure. Within the UK the RAF operate such a chamber at the Centre for Aviation Medicine, RAF Henlow.

An alternative technique is to replace oxygen with nitrogen, thus reducing FiO2 to mimic a specific altitude (normobaric hypoxia, or NH). This technique is readily available and widely used by sports scientists to test altitude training protocols. Effectively, all that is required is a sealed room and it is therefore easier for investigators (or unwell subjects) to move from the chamber to the lab outside. The RAF do this training using an aircrew mask and gas supply rather than making a sealed room hypoxic.

Finally, the other option is to locate the laboratory at HA in the real-world environment. Within Europe there are a variety of mountain huts at altitudes as high as 4,559m, some of which can be easily reached by cable car, although others are more difficult to access, though they can be serviced by helicopters to carry kit and personnel to.

DHAULAGIRI Research Expedition is conducted by the British military's Royal Centre for Defence Medicine (Academic Department of Military Anaesthesia and Critical Care and Academic Department of Military Medicine) in conjunction with researchers from Leeds Beckett University's Institute for Sports Physical Activity Leisure and Oxford University.

The research projects include:

- Study 1   Acclimation and acclimatisation: The effects of exercise under normobaric hypoxic conditions.
- Study 2   Biomechanical changes in walking and balance at altitude.
- Study 3   Application of apnoeic training and physiological adaptations to altitude.
- Study 4   Appetite responses during high-altitude expeditions.
- Study 5   Monitoring of heart rate and rhythm during the ascent to extreme altitude.
- Study 6   The investigation of the adaptation of the heart and lungs to high altitude.
- Study 7   The use of brain natriuretic hormone as a marker for high-altitude illness.

Source:
www.dhaulagiri2016.com/medical-research.

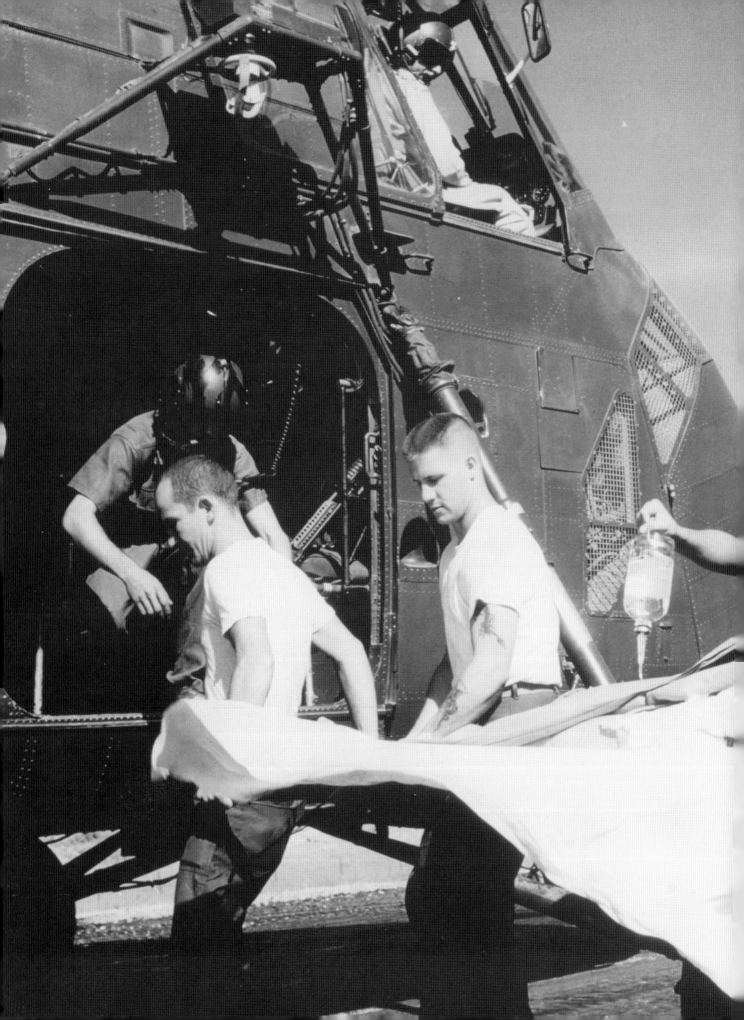

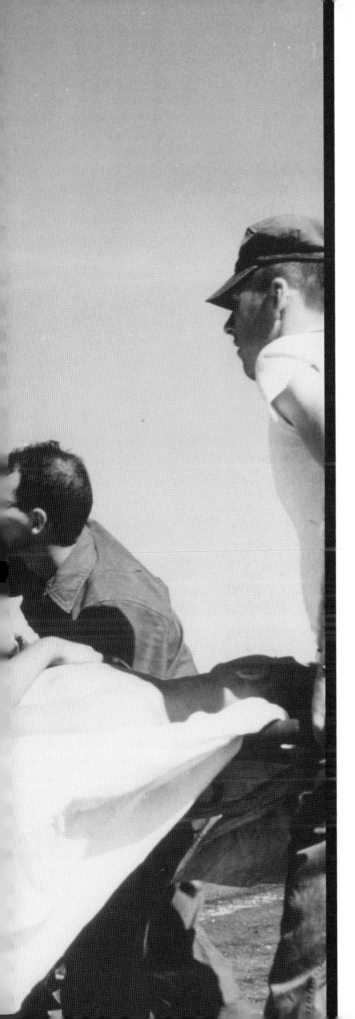

Chapter Five

Vascular surgery

The Korean War was a watershed in terms of vascular surgery. The ability to use penicillin as antibiotic cover, combined with new blood transfusion techniques and innovative arterial/venous patches led to the widespread reconstruction of arteries, veins and lymphatic vessels.

OPPOSITE A US Marine casualty receives dextrose as he is carried onto a waiting Sikorsky H-34 helicopter for transfer to the USS *Repose*, Vietnam, 4 April 1966. *(US Navy photo)*

79

VASCULAR SURGERY

Over the course of centuries, the history of blood transfusion and vascular surgery has been persistently controversial. From the ancient Greeks, who first suggested the possibility of blood transfusions, to 20th-century notions of social Darwinism, cultural, racial and religious belief systems have attached an almost mythical symbolism to the circulatory system and life-giving properties of blood. Scientific discoveries such as the use of sodium citrate and refrigeration to prolong the storage lifespan of blood, separation of blood plasma, the introduction of mobile transfusion units, identification of the rhesus factor, and significant advances in blood and tissue typing in the 1930s, were frequently overshadowed by a pervading ethos of nationalistic racial dogma. French doctors conducting research into blood typing during this era, for example, confidently proclaimed that people living in Western Europe, who were predominantly A-positive, were far superior to those living in Eastern Europe, who mainly had B-negative blood. One went so far as to suggest that people with A-positive blood took less time to defecate than their B-negative counterparts! Furthermore, the linking of dubious blood-typing characteristics with ridiculous notions of racial superiority did much to fuel the flames of fascism.

In 1936, during the Spanish Civil War, following in the footsteps of Dr Frederic Durán-Jordà, who established a blood bank and transfusion service in Barcelona, Canadian-born Professor Norman Bethune formed a large network of mobile transfusion teams from his base in Madrid. Covering a territory of over 90km, he successfully supplied blood to front-line troops throughout the conflict. Innovations in the treatment of war wounds also emerged from 1936 onwards, with Barcelona's Professor Josep Trueta introducing a new regime of wound debridement and aftercare. This included early surgery, rigorous wound cleaning, excision of dead tissue, wound drainage and the immobilisation of injured limbs within a closed cast of plaster of Paris.

Yet while the Spanish experience prompted numerous advances in vascular surgery, elsewhere – particularly in Germany – some doctors were vilified for performing blood transfusions. Jewish doctor Hans Serelman, for example, performed a dramatic and impromptu blood transfusion in his own private surgery. In order to save a patient's

BELOW Diagram of blood grouping.

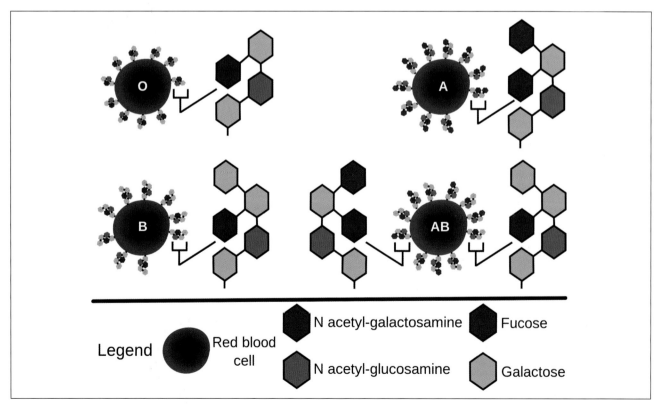

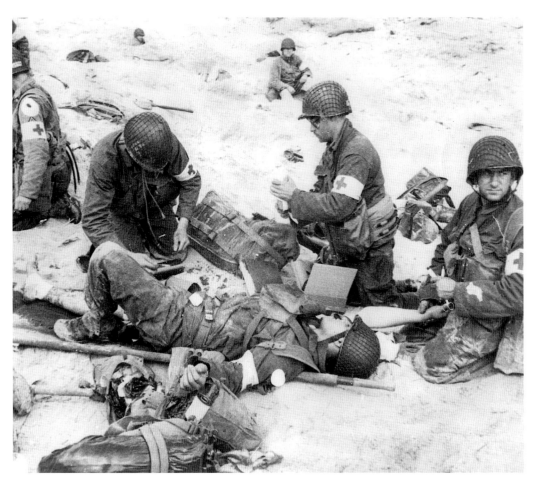

life, he excised his own artery and transfused his patient with his own blood. His patient survived, but doctor Serelman was tried, condemned and imprisoned for tainting pure Aryan German blood. Problems associated with blood transfusions also surfaced in the USA during the Second World War, because white US soldiers injured in combat flatly refused to receive transfusions of African-American blood. Consequently, US military medics were forced to establish white and black blood banks.

British military doctors, meanwhile, adopted a more pragmatic approach to the subject of transfusions. Following on from successes achieved in casualty clearing stations on the Western Front during the First World War, whole blood was routinely given to casualties suffering from haemorrhagic shock from 1939 onwards. British Red Cross workers had established the first volunteer blood donor scheme in 1921 and British Army officials opened the first blood storage depot in Bristol in 1938.

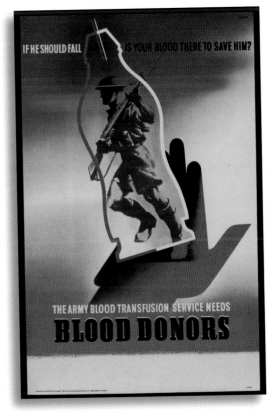

IF HE SHOULD FALL   IS YOUR BLOOD THERE TO SAVE HIM?

THE ARMY BLOOD TRANSFUSION SERVICE NEEDS
BLOOD DONORS

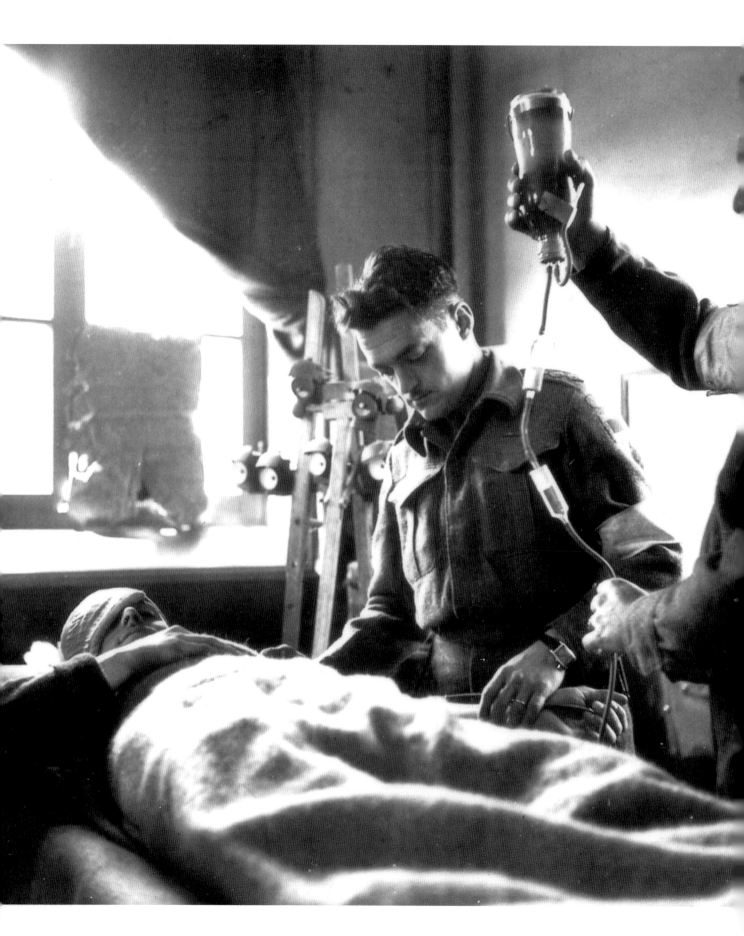

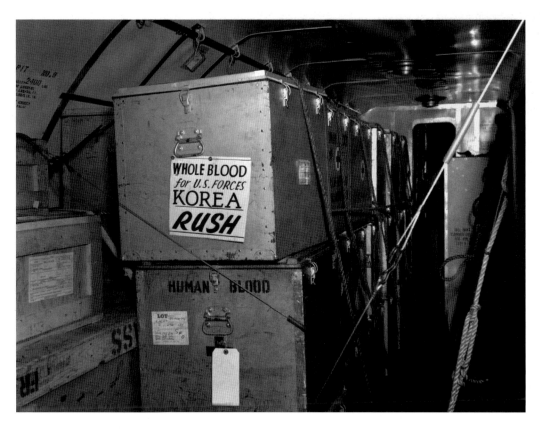

OPPOSITE A British Army doctor tends to an injured soldier in Normandy while a medical orderly holds a blood flask for transfusion. (USNA)

LEFT Whole blood supplies, Korea. Blood for use in the Korean War was stored and distributed from military base hospitals in Japan. The replacement of bottles with plastic bags to store and transport blood and blood products was an important innovation, reducing the incidence of haemolysis and freeing up more space on aircraft to increase the volume of blood supplies delivered. (Shutterstock)

With infrastructures for the distribution of blood firmly in place, military physicians were able to safely transfuse casualties throughout the Second World War. Mobile blood units with storage facilities, which the troops affectionately nicknamed 'vampire vans', also travelled to forward areas when necessary to obtain donations from fit, healthy Army personnel. However, whereas British Army medics favoured transfusions of whole blood for the injured, US forces preferred to administer plasma. This trend continued during the Korean War.

As a tool for resuscitation plasma was very useful, especially when whole blood was unavailable. Yet serum hepatitis could easily be contracted from plasma infusions because of problems associated with sterilisation methods. In fact, most of the US plasma used during the first year of the Korean War was completely untreated. Not surprisingly cases of hepatitis following plasma transfusion soared from 7.5% during the Second World War, to 21% by the end of 1951. To counteract substantial failings in sterilisation, plasma was treated with ultraviolet light, but cases of hepatitis continued to rise. Eventually the US Army designated its 35th Station Hospital in Kyoto as a hepatitis

centre and issued an official directive in 1953 prohibiting the use of plasma to correct hypovolaemia during resuscitation unless other intravenous fluids were unavailable.

Despite these significant problems the Korean War became renowned for major advances in transfusion techniques and vascular surgery. Pioneer Army surgeon Michael De Bakey led the way in vascular reconstruction, repairing aortic aneurisms and

BELOW 'Prevent Hepatitis' poster. (US Air Force photo)

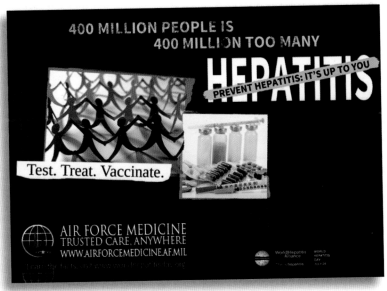

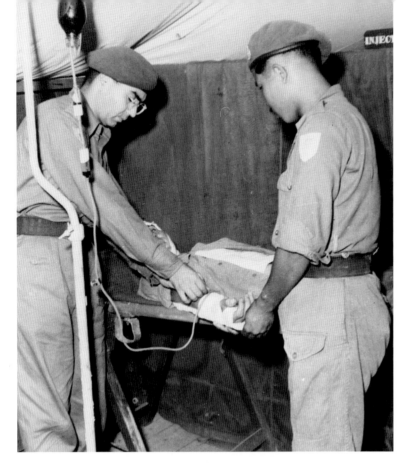

blocked carotid arteries by grafting frozen blood vessels on to damaged segments of the arterial system. He also developed a roller pump, which became an integral part of cardiopulmonary bypass machines, and by the end of the war had devised Dacron tubing to repair injured or diseased blood vessels.

The combination of these revolutionary techniques prompted a new era in cardio thoracic surgery. Under his guidance MASH became the norm and improvements in vascular surgery dramatically increased casualty survival rates. Indeed, those who were admitted to a MASH unit had a 95% chance of surviving their injuries. Moreover, the widespread use of penicillin and sulphonamides enabled surgeons to perform complicated vascular surgery without the risk of secondary post-operative infections. These surgical improvements were not confined to the field of abdominal and cardio thoracic surgery. Patients suffering from septic shock due to haemorrhagic fever, for instance, were given dialysis to correct renal insufficiency using newly developed artificial kidneys. Moreover, vascular reconstruction of limbs reduced the need for amputations from 36% during the Second World War to 13% in the Korean War and 8% during the Vietnam Conflict.

The severity of Korean winters took its toll on combat troops, however, and veterans continued to experience vascular problems long after the cessation of hostilities. These included peripheral nerve damage, the likelihood of skin cancer in areas previously affected by frostbite, chronic pain in hands and feet and osteoarthritis.[1] Those who served near, or were involved with, nuclear testing sites also developed latent and frequently fatal complications of military service.

In terms of vascular surgery, physicians

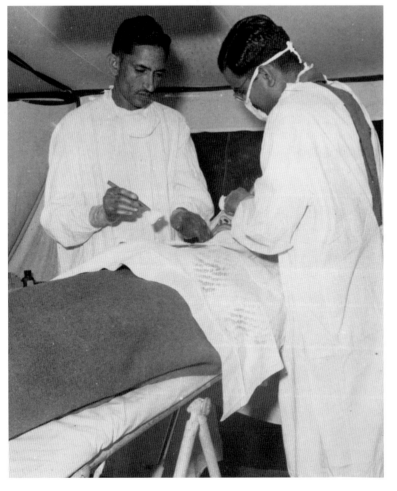

working with US medical services in Vietnam generally continued the success of their predecessors. Perhaps unsurprisingly, many surgeons recruited from civilian hospitals were ill prepared for combat surgery, since even the busiest civilian surgical department bore no comparison to the chaotic and frenetic pace of work which was commonplace in military combat zones. Neither were they prepared for the unrelenting and disturbing scenes of severely injured casualties – where in some instances, bodies were barely recognisable. Blood-splattered operating theatres were constantly in use and stemming the blood flow in casualties who had been blasted by ballistic weapons was an ongoing challenge. Discovering the source of bleeding was a frantic race against the clock, because patients could exsanguinate rapidly. On a practical skill level, civilian surgeons working on the front line were often criticised for their adherence to specialism and for making small opening incisions. The latter technique worked well in straightforward civilian surgical procedures but was not appropriate for wounds caused by gunshots and weapon blasts, which needed larger, more expansive excisions. Shrapnel or other debris could be pushed far into the body by sheer ballistic force and a small incision left little room for exploring wounds. The likelihood of debris emerging several hours after initial wounding also ensured that delayed wound closure became a feature of military surgery in Vietnam. Wounds were left open for a period of at least four days, sometimes up to ten days, covered by a loose sterile gauze dressing. This allowed time for swelling to reduce, bleeding to slow down and any remaining debris to surface. If there was any sign of infection, then antibiotic treatment was commenced before wound closure. As the war progressed, wound dressings were infused with antiseptics or antibiotics and applied directly to post-operative wounds.

The longevity of hostilities in Vietnam prompted several medical research projects. Clinical laboratories were attached to MASH units, and microbiologists were deployed to gather data and perform forensic analysis. These highly skilled health professionals were instrumental in reducing the numbers of soldiers suffering from disease and non-battle injuries from 774 per 1,000 personnel during the Korean Conflict, to 419 per 1,000 personnel in Vietnam.[2] In addition, microbiologists were responsible for screening patients and identifying the presence of communicable diseases such as malaria, parasitic infestations, tuberculosis and the plague. Wound cultures were routinely tested to determine the presence of bacteria, and to ascertain bacterial sensitivity to antibiotics. In the hot, humid environment infectious diseases spread rapidly and in one year, between 1966 and 1967, 70% of hospital admissions were due to communicable diseases.[3] This situation impacted considerably on the ability to obtain donors of fresh whole blood from within the ranks. Known by this stage as the 'walking

BELOW Open heart surgery aboard USS *Repose* steaming off the coast of Vietnam in November 1966. The patient is attached to the Baylor-Bell heart and lung machine. *(US Navy photo)*

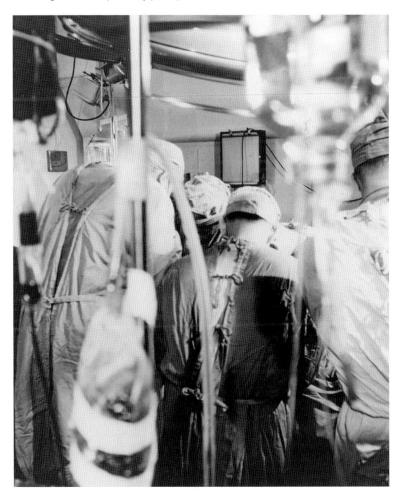

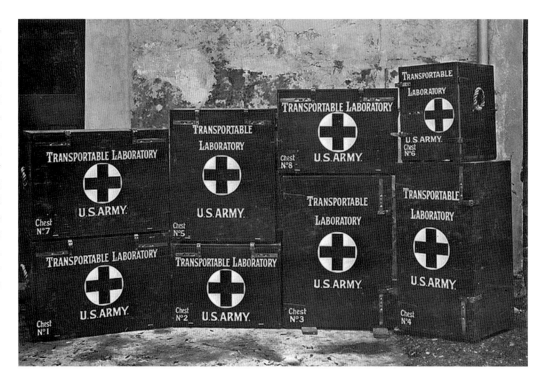

blood bank', troops were frequently asked to donate blood for incoming wounded, but increasing numbers were prevented from doing so because of associated problems of pathogen transference. Moreover, the ease of illicit drug availability fuelled growing addiction levels among troops in Vietnam, which further contributed to the paucity of blood donors.

Vascular surgeons continued to develop their skills, substituting non-blood products for resuscitation when necessary, and new techniques in radiography greatly assisted their surgical interventions. Field medical facilities usually contained at least one X-ray machine, and technology originally developed to improve night vision for troops eventually produced image intensifiers for use in the operating theatre. By the end of the Vietnam War there was also a growing recognition that the deployment of some surgical specialists in forward medical units could be of immense value.

In the early 1980s, referring to medical lessons learned as a result of the British Falkland Islands Campaign, senior surgeon P.S. London stated:

To surgeons brought up to technical elaboration in familiar, protective and more leisurely conditions, the needs of war surgery are likely to be strange and alarming [. . .] It is, therefore, imperative that all surgeons in training should become familiar with what is essential and what can be done in far from ideal conditions. Teachers of surgery have a duty not only to equip themselves with necessary knowledge but to see to it whenever possible their apprentices and journeymen make use of the safe and well proven methods that 'burn no boats'. For these purposes the need is for surgeons of body-wide competence, not narrow skills; and these are in civilian as well as military surgical activities, because the limb mangled in a road accident has much in common with that mangled by a mine or other destructive weapon of war. How many surgical teachers can say that they have adequately equipped themselves and their trainees and how many that have not done so will at once seek to make good their deficiencies? If it is asked whether there is a place for surgical specialists in forward units, the answer is yes: neurosurgeons and oral and dental surgeons have proved their value, if not in their proper tasks, then by acting as sorters, organisers and resuscitators.[4]

Dr Rick Jolly, in charge of the field hospital in Ajax Bay, described the range of emotions experienced by combat surgeons as they performed vascular surgery in the Falklands:

The young man was lying on a stretcher, shocked and shivering, with wide staring eyes, his blood-soaked clothing cut from his pale but well-muscled body as the Fenwal blood bags drained into each arm. Chief McKinley, the transfusion technician, had two more bags of the chilled blood warming in his shirt pockets, grimacing as he tried to hide his discomfort. Four units later, Captain Y was on the table in theatre. Bill McGregor was first knife, with Charles Batty assisting. A bold slash, and Bill was through a right paramedian incision and into the abdominal cavity. A dark red clot flopped into the wound as the surgeon's fingers searched for the bleeding point. 'There it is . . .,' said Bill quietly, and we all craned our necks to see. The right lobe of the liver had been gouged by a bullet. More clots were scooped out as another assistant pulled harder on the retractor that lifted the rib cage up and away from Bill's line of sight. Some fancy needlework with deep catgut sutures followed; several folded gauzes made of oxycellulose were then packed in, and the liver laceration was repaired. But the bleeding continued, and Bill was despairing. He had discovered that there was another hole beneath all this mess, but this one was the vena cava, the wide-bore main vein that carries blood from the limbs and kidneys back to the heart. This was really major-league stuff. Malcolm Jowitt whispered his encouragement, and Bill loaded a round-bodied needle with catgut and tried again. After a tense moment as he felt his way to the bottom of the deep, dark hole before him, he brought the needle holder out and tied a surgical knot. This time the bleeding stopped. At the head of the table, Major Jowitt looked well pleased with his surgeon as Bill and Charles packed the recesses of the hole with more oxycellulose, and then closed the belly. John Y not only survived, but later underwent and passed Special Air Service Selection, and then completed his Army career with 22 SAS in Hereford.[5]

While military surgeons debated the issue of general versus specialist skills on the battlefield, approaches to combat surgery began to shift in the direction of simply limiting the immediate damage caused by injuries until further expertise was available. This policy of damage-control surgery, which aimed to stabilise a casualty before reaching an intensive-therapy unit, was firmly in place by 1995. Immediate treatment focused on preventing catastrophic haemorrhage, performing resuscitative measures and protecting organs within the abdominal cavity. Combined with damage-control resuscitation, damage-control surgery is now normal practice within combat zones.

BELOW A casualty from HMS *Sheffield* is rushed to HMS *Hermes* on 4 May 1982 after the frigate was struck and set on fire by an Exocet missile launched from an Argentinian Super Etendard aircraft. *(IWM FKD534)*

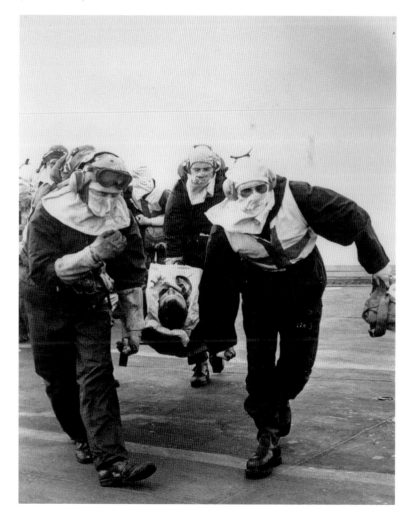

FLUIDS COMMONLY USED IN RESUSCITATION

Blood components:
- Whole blood
- Packed red blood cells
- Plasma
- Freeze-dried plasma
- Platelets

Non-blood fluids used for resuscitation:
- Normal saline
- Dextrose/dextran
- Hartmann's solution contains a mixture of electrolytes – sodium chloride, sodium lactate, potassium chloride and calcium dihydrate. Occasionally this mixture is fortified with extra potassium chloride.
- Ringer's solution is designed to correct isotonic dehydration and mimic the components of plasma. It contains water, sodium chloride, potassium chloride and calcium chloride dihydrate.

Initially military surgeons were extremely reluctant to perform limited surgical interventions. Writing of his experiences in Iraq during Operation Iraqi Freedom, Operation Enduring Freedom and in Afghanistan, Harvard graduate Atul Gawande MD asserted:

It is a system that took some getting used to. Surgeons at every level initially tended to hold on to their patients, either believing that they could provide definitive care themselves or not trusting that the next level could do so. According to statistics from Walter Reed, during the first few months of the war, it took an injured soldier an average of eight days to go from the battlefield to a US care facility. Gradually, however, surgeons have embraced the wisdom of the system. The average time from battlefield to arrival in the US is now less than four days. In Vietnam it was 45 days. Today, military surgical strategy aims for damage control, not definitive repair, unless it can be done quickly. Teams pack off liver injuries, staple off perforated bowels, wash out dirty wounds – whatever

BELOW A German soldier puts on a tourniquet during a military exercise. Since catastrophic haemorrhage is the leading cause of battlefield deaths, tourniquet application is an essential skill.
(Shutterstock)

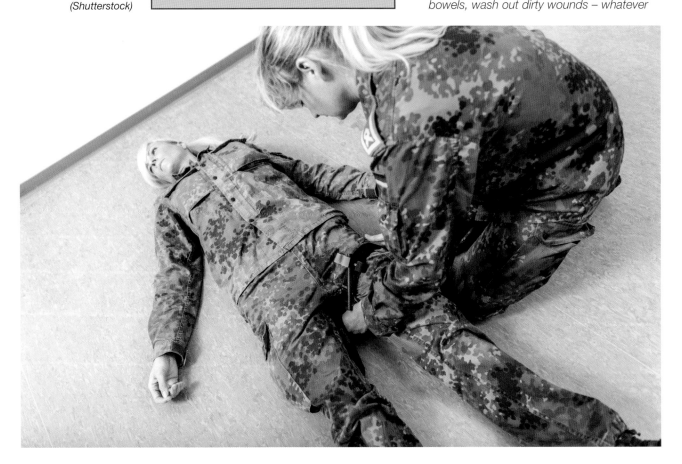

*is necessary to stop bleeding and control
contamination without allowing the patient
to lose body temperature or become
coagulopathic. Surgeons seek to limit
surgery to two hours or less, and then ship
the patient off to a combat support hospital
[. . .] the next level of care. Abdomens can
be left open, laparotomy pads left in, bowel
unanastomosed, the patient paralysed,
sedated, ventilated. For this approach to be
successful, however, control of airspace and
major roadways and establishment of the
next level hospital (achieved early in Iraq but
delayed in Afghanistan) are essential.[6]*

Mortality rates from battlefield injuries continued
to fall in the decades since Korea, but the
overriding cause of preventable deaths has
remained constant. Catastrophic haemorrhage
was, and still is, the leading cause of death
on the battlefield. Compressible and non-
compressible bleeding remains the biggest
challenge for combat medics.

Increased use of tourniquets and newly
developed haemostatic products have made a
considerable impact in improving haemorrhage
survival rates, but non-extremity blood loss still
poses a severe problem. Furthermore, combat
casualties are frequently injured in remote areas
or difficult terrains, where fresh whole blood and
other resuscitative infusions are either in short
supply or non-existent. Some blood loss can
usually be stemmed by external compression
on pressure points or directly on to bleeding
wounds, but others, particularly those of the
truncal area are difficult to manage. Gaping
wounds are usually packed with combat
gauze infused with haemostatic agents, which
accelerate the clotting process, and calcium
is sometimes administered for its haemostatic
properties. For external wounds pressure is also
applied for a period of three minutes. QuikClot
and Chitosan, which are formulated from shrimp
shells, have proved their efficacy as haemostatic
agents in recent conflicts. Non-absorbable
haemostatic expandable sponges (XSTAT),
consisting of approximately 92 discoid sponges
impregnated with Chitosan have also achieved
dramatic results. Once injected into the wound
cavity, the sponges expand from 4.5mm disks
to 40mm tubes when in contact with blood,

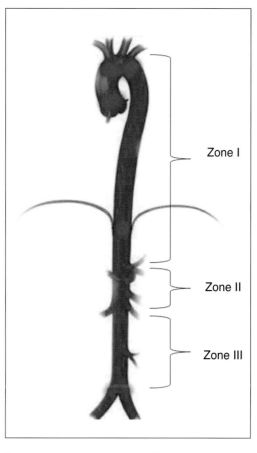

LEFT Diagram of
aorta zones.

Zone I

Zone II

Zone III

thus tamponading bleeding. Sponges have
radiopaque markers to facilitate retrieval and
are particularly useful for wounds situated in the
groin or armpit.[7]

In recent years resuscitative endovascular
balloon occlusion devices (REBOA), inserted
into the aorta, have proved extremely valuable
in controlling excessive bleeding in cases of
non-compressible truncal haemorrhaging.

The idea of using balloon-occlusive
techniques to control bleeding was first mooted
in Korea. However, the notion was shelved
because of the fear of causing permanent
ischaemia to vital organs, and substantial
difficulties associated with training and
technology. Modern medical advances and
the ongoing need to provide life-saving pre-
hospital care for exsanguinating casualties has
prompted more research into the possible use
of balloon-occlusive treatments. Using arterial
cannulation procedures, devices are usually
inserted through a sheath into the femoral
artery, with or without the use of a guide wire.
Balloon inflation in the supraceliac aorta acts in
a similar way to an aortic cross clamp placed

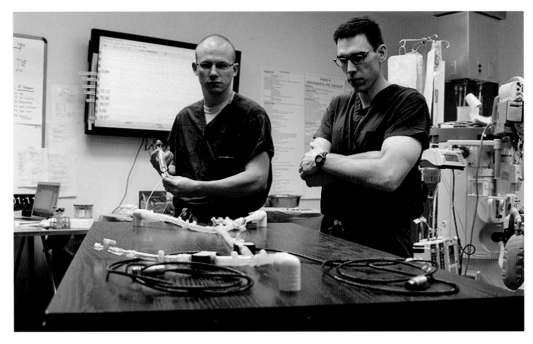

RIGHT Bench-testing of resuscitative endovascular balloon occlusion of the aorta catheters. *(US Air Force)*

BELOW Diagram of endovascular balloon occlusive devices.

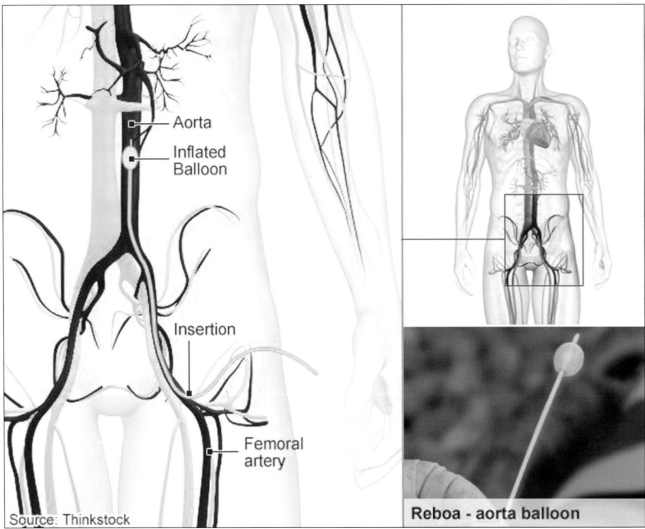

Aorta

Inflated Balloon

Insertion

Femoral artery

Source: Thinkstock

Reboa - aorta balloon

during resuscitative thoracotomy and inflation time is limited to 60 minutes to prevent death of abdominal contents. When inflated in the infra-renal aorta, the balloon controls bleeding in the pelvic area. Critics of the procedure have argued that arterial cannulation is too difficult for some pre-hospital medics to perform, especially under duress. They also point out that significant risk of ischaemia is also problematic in patients where occlusion is prolonged. Yet early research findings have demonstrated improved civilian casualty survival rates using balloon occlusion devices compared to resuscitative thoracotomy. Medical research is ongoing in this area and it is possible that resuscitative endovascular balloon occlusion will be the treatment of choice for some cases of haemorrhage control in the future. Balloon-occlusive procedures are not used in the UK military, however, because of difficulties associated with maintaining cleanliness of the insertion site during evacuation to a field hospital, and the fact that it would be virtually impossible to insert the kit in a moving aircraft.[8]

Furthermore, as Colonel Harvey Pynn RAMC has asserted:

> REBOA is currently unproven and there are less invasive means of stopping blood flow to the lower part of the body, such as abdominal tourniquets. Certainly, the latter is easier to apply. As yet there have been no studies comparing REBOA with external non-invasive devices. Until this is clarified there is no place for REBOA in the PHEC [pre-hospital emergency care] space in the UK military. It is also worth noting that REBOA should only be placed for relatively short periods, else critical ischaemia will set in. Uncontrollable, non-compressible haemorrhage still needs a surgeon in the military environment – another reason not to launch into using REBOA.[9]

Added to physical and practical applications to stem blood loss, systemic medications such as TXA, which inhibits the breakdown of blood clots, play a significant role in preventing deaths from haemorrhage. A multinational Clinical Randomisation of an Antifibrinolytic in Significant Haemorrhage -2 (CRASH-2) study

RECOMMENDATIONS FOR REMOTE DAMAGE-CONTROL RESUSCITATION

- Rapidly identify patient with significant haemorrhage.
- As soon as possible (ideally at point of injury): obtain mechanical haemorrhage control with haemostatic gauzes and/or extremity tourniquet and commence resuscitation with reconstituted freeze-dried plasma and administer Tranexamic acid (if available).
- Transition to (in order of preference): whole blood, 1:1:1 plasma: Red Blood Cells: platelets, 1:1 plasma: Red Blood Cells.
- Reassess limb tourniquet every 2 hours and convert to a haemostatic or pressure dressing, if able.
- Minimise use of crystalloids and artificial colloids.
- Do not administer Tranexamic acid >3 hours after injury.
- For patients without traumatic brain injury and minimal expected pre-hospital transport time, permissive hypotension is safe. However, there is insufficient data for a recommendation for patients with traumatic brain injury or expected transport delay.

Source: R. Chang, B.J. Eastridge and J.B. Holcombe, 'Tactical Combat Casualty Care: Transitioning Battlefield Lessons Learned to other Austere Environments', *Wilderness and Environmental Medicine*, 28 (2017), S124–S134.

randomised > 20,000 trauma patients at risk for haemorrhage to TXA vs placebo and found that TXA reduced all-cause mortality (14.5% vs 16%) and exsanguination-associated mortality (4.9% vs 5.7%).[10] Further analysis and trials revealed that the effects of TXA were time dependent, and most effective when administered to casualties within an hour of injury (5.3% vs 7.7%), with a lesser effect when given between 1 and 3 hours (4.8% vs 6.1%) and an increased risk of exsanguination when given after 3 hours

(4.4% vs 3.1%). Moreover, the drug was shown to improve survival rates in 231 massively transfused (>10 RBC units in 24 hours) combat casualties.[11] A study of 414 patients who underwent massive transfusions in a CSH in Baghdad, Iraq, found that the mortality rate was 27%, whereas in Bastion it was 4%. A further study which examined the use of TXA in war-wounded, massively transfused patients, reported a 24-hour mortality rate of 9.6%. The results of all these studies concluded that all in-hospital mortality rates were low.[12]

In addition to stemming the blood flow in casualties suffering from catastrophic haemorrhage, combat medics also need to replace the blood already lost. Clinical decisions for massive blood transfusions are determined by the extent of blood loss and by vital signs. For instance, if systolic blood pressure is below 90 and heart rate above 110 beats per minute, then transfusion is normally necessary. Casualties requiring massive transfusions have usually sustained blast injuries, penetrating wounds or traumatic amputations.[13] Whole

blood is usually considered to be the best transfusion option in this situation, but resuscitative measures are often dependent on combat conditions and environment. During the Falklands Campaign:

Resuscitation was carried out using Hartmann's solution, and for burns polygeline, dextran 70 and dextran 110. Much of the blood was drawn from the troops a week or ten days before battle and from fit convalescents before they were evacuated. 3 Commando Brigade provided 1,300 bags of blood and it was found that three per cent of the blood groups had been wrongly recorded. Two batches of nearly 400 bags were also sent from the United Kingdom. Although citrate-phosphate-dextrose solution allows blood to be used up to six weeks after it was drawn, little was available. Field conditions did not allow cross-matching and group O blood was given; from the infusion of more than 200 bags there was only one mild

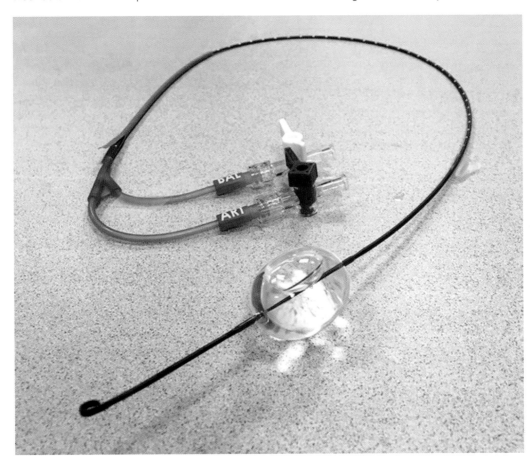

RIGHT Freeze-dried plasma. *(US Air Force)*

reaction. In all only 600 bags were used – 18 per cent of what was available – because casualties were fewer than expected. In the hospital ship Uganda *an average of five bags was used for each patient; one man with a torn inferior vena cava was given 38. In addition to resuscitation when necessary, the wounded received tetanus toxoid and penicillin, with sulphadiazine and metronidazole for wounds of the head and gentamycin and metronidazole for wounds of the belly. Morphine was given intravenously when needed.*[14]

Whole blood (and other blood products such as platelets or plasma) was usually the transfusion choice for casualty resuscitation, but by the mid-1980s problems associated with pathogen transmission in blood transfusion came to the fore again; the HIV/AIDS epidemic threatened to eclipse all blood-transmitted pathogens that had gone before. US and NATO military medics were quick to introduce blood screening procedures from 1985 onwards, but the heightened risk of blood contamination associated with HIV and other sexually transmitted diseases loomed large for decades to come. In some instances, an overriding fear of blood pathogens created a shift in clinical practice, with US combat medics frequently using artificial colloids as replacement fluids in hypovolaemia. Nevertheless, clinical data which later emerged from resuscitation practices in Operation Iraqi Freedom and Operation Enduring Freedom clearly demonstrated that survival rates were improved when casualties were transfused with plasma and platelets instead of artificial colloids.[15]

NATO allies, particularly France and Germany, have achieved considerable success in using freeze-dried plasma (FDP) in forward remote terrains where logistical restrictions have precluded the use of other blood products. Given to troops (especially special forces) to carry along with separate phials of sterile water, it can be mixed quickly and can replace blood loss in an emergency. Manufactured in France, Germany and South Africa, FDP is currently safer to use because methods of deactivating pathogens were updated during the 1990s. US forces have been slow to adopt this trend, however, because

BENEFITS OF LOW TITER GROUP O WHOLE BLOOD FOR HAEMORRHAGIC SHOCK

Efficacy – The cold-stored platelets (PLTs) provide improved haemostasis compared with room temperature PLTs

Whole blood is a more concentrated product that contains a smaller quantity of anticoagulant and additive solution than an equal amount of conventional components

Safety – Reduced risk of haemolysis from the low titer minor incompatible plasma compared to the risk from untitered minor incompatible plasma or PLTs

■ Reduced risk of bacterial contamination compared to room-temperature-stored PLTs

■ Long-standing safety record with over a million units transfused in combat and civilian settings

Logistic – Increased access to PLTs for both pre-hospital and early in-hospital resuscitations

■ Simplifies the logistics of the resuscitation and accelerates the provision of all blood components needed to treat haemorrhagic shock.

Source: M.H. Yaser, A.P. Cap and P.C. Spinella, 'Raising the Standards on Whole Blood', *Journal of Trauma Acute Care Surgery*, 86 (6) (28 December 2017), 1.

of previous experience of disease transmission via plasma in Korea and Vietnam. Scientific research aims to redress this problem and future developments include the possibility of freeze-drying a soldier's plasma, to be stored for his own personal use (thus removing the risk of transfusion infection and eliminating the possibility of a reaction). Stem cell treatment is also a futuristic development. In the summer of 2018, the US military officially approved emergency use of French FDP, while US Food and Drug Agency surveys reveal growing evidence that FDP saves lives on the battlefield.

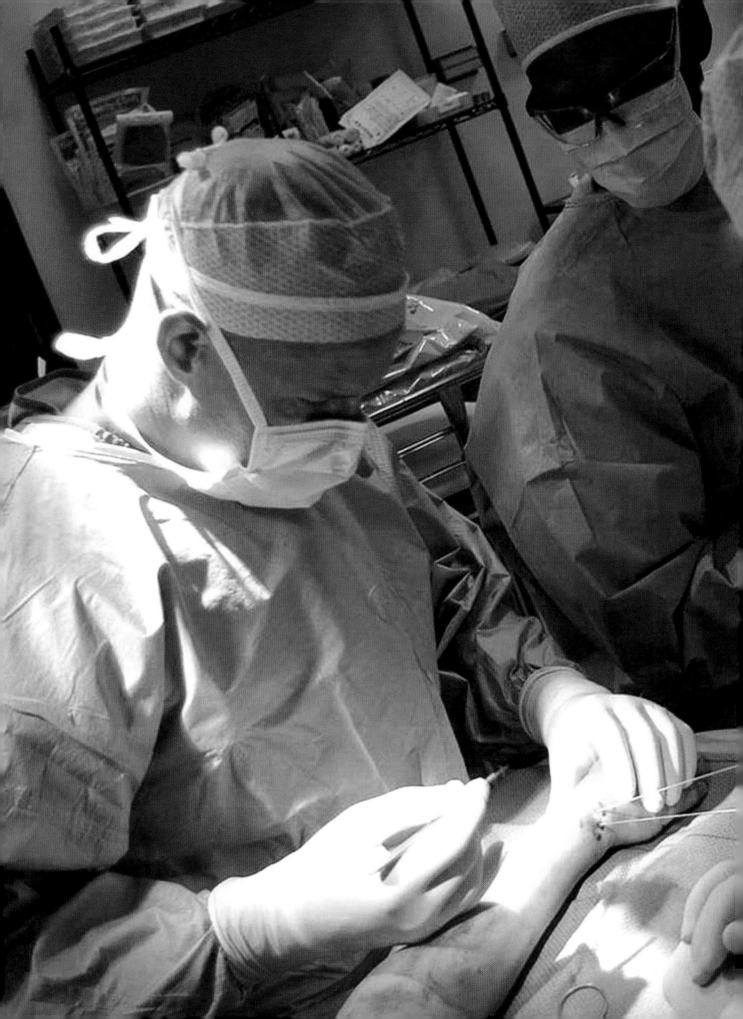

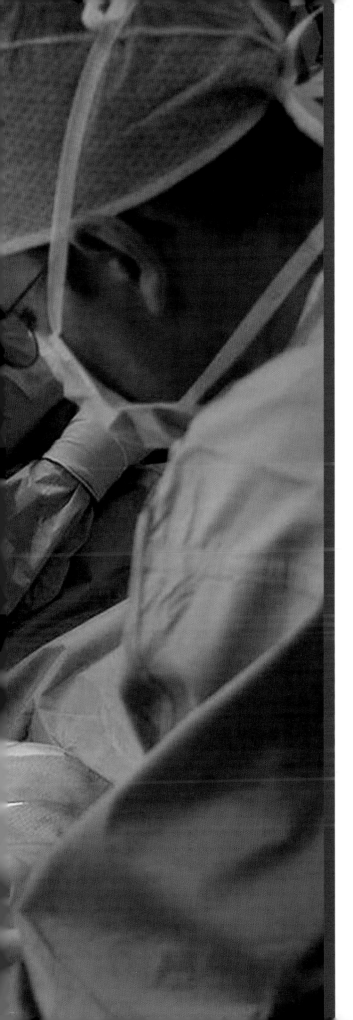

Chapter Six

Orthopaedic surgery

Orthopaedic surgeons were no strangers to war wounds. Yet the blasts from improvised explosive devices (IEDs) in Iraq and Afghanistan produced mangled limbs and multiple compound fractures on an unprecedented scale. The complexity of these wounds fostered a closer relationship between orthopaedic specialists and plastic surgeons.

OPPOSITE US Air Force orthopaedic surgeons at work. *(US Air Force photo)*

In terms of combat medicine, rudimentary surgery involving bones, muscles, nerves and skin can be traced to Ancient Greece and Egypt. Even in the days of Hippocrates basic amputations were performed on the battlefield, and rudimentary prosthetics developed. But despite the undoubted usefulness in dealing with combat injuries, for many centuries orthopaedic surgery was considered the lowest of the low by mainstream medical men; summarily dismissed as being the most simple and basic of all forms of medical intervention. Physicians aiming to build a reputation in the world during the 19th century believed that little skill was needed to conduct bone surgery, arguing that all that was required was brute force. It was around this time that physicians in England (often referred to as 'quacks'), concerned with raising their status, decided to adopt the title 'doctor', because this was the title awarded to Oxbridge-educated men who had studied to become doctors of philosophy. By assuming the highest title in the land, physicians automatically raised their profile and sought to establish professional specialisms. But orthopaedics was still relegated to the margins of medicine. Indeed, by the late 19th century men preoccupied with the medical or surgical treatment of the musculoskeletal system were merely referred to as 'bone setters'. Childhood cases of rickets, limbs affected by tuberculosis as well as broken bones and congenital defects of the skeletal structure, were all treated either conservatively or surgically by bone setters.

But during the First World War, particularly between 1914 and 1916, compound fractures of the femur (broken thigh bones which also broke through the skin) were the most common and lethal of all battlefield injuries. Over 80% of all soldiers who sustained these injuries died. The friction caused by bone ends rubbing together caused extreme shock and haemorrhage and soldiers usually exsanguinated before reaching casualty clearing stations. Attempts to immobilise these fractures by supporting the injured leg with a rifle or pole tied to the thigh were often futile. Consequently, soldiers were frequently forced to carry out life-saving amputations on their injured pals using kit knives and improvised tourniquets. However, this situation changed significantly in 1916 when the Thomas splint was introduced to the Western Front. Originally designed by Hugh Owen Thomas for treating tuberculosis patients, the splint provided support for leg fractures by means of parallel poles fixed to a metal ring situated at the upper end of the thigh, supportive canvas slings could be attached to the poles and a system of traction, pulleys, cords and weights successfully immobilised the limb. Thomas's nephew, surgeon Robert Jones, brought the splints to base hospitals and the eminent surgeon Colonel Henry Gray ensured their widespread use. According to Jones, the splints could be used for all fractured femurs, severe fractures near the knee joint or upper tibia and in some patients with severe flesh wounds to the thigh. It could not be applied, however, if open wounds were too close to the upper ring of the splint. Surgeons needed to be careful to align fractures to prevent disability and injured legs were normally splinted for around three months. Moreover, applications of Thomas splints had an enormous impact on the Western Front, reducing death rates due to compound fractures of the femur from 80% to under 20%, and orthopaedics emerged as a distinct and valuable medical specialism. Furthermore, as over 40,000 British amputee soldiers returned home from war, a prosthetic industry quickly emerged to meet the growing demand for artificial limbs.

Orthopaedics assumed centre stage once more during the Spanish Civil War. Barcelona was subjected to over 340 air raids and the treatment of Spanish casualties revolutionised medical opinion in Britain and elsewhere. Professor Trueta, chief of a large surgical unit in Barcelona, claimed that Spanish experience had shown that unless injuries received 'on-the-spot' skilled attention, subsequent treatment was often useless. Advising the British government in October 1939, Trueta argued that skilled surgical teams needed to be in the centre of all major cities to treat victims of aerial bombardment, and at the front line of combat zones. He also described his five-step wound treatment and reduction of fractures; to the extent of showing medical teams his collection of photographs of limbs encased in plaster casts stained with severely yellow or green wound exudate. Despite outward appearances these pus-forming wounds, hidden beneath a

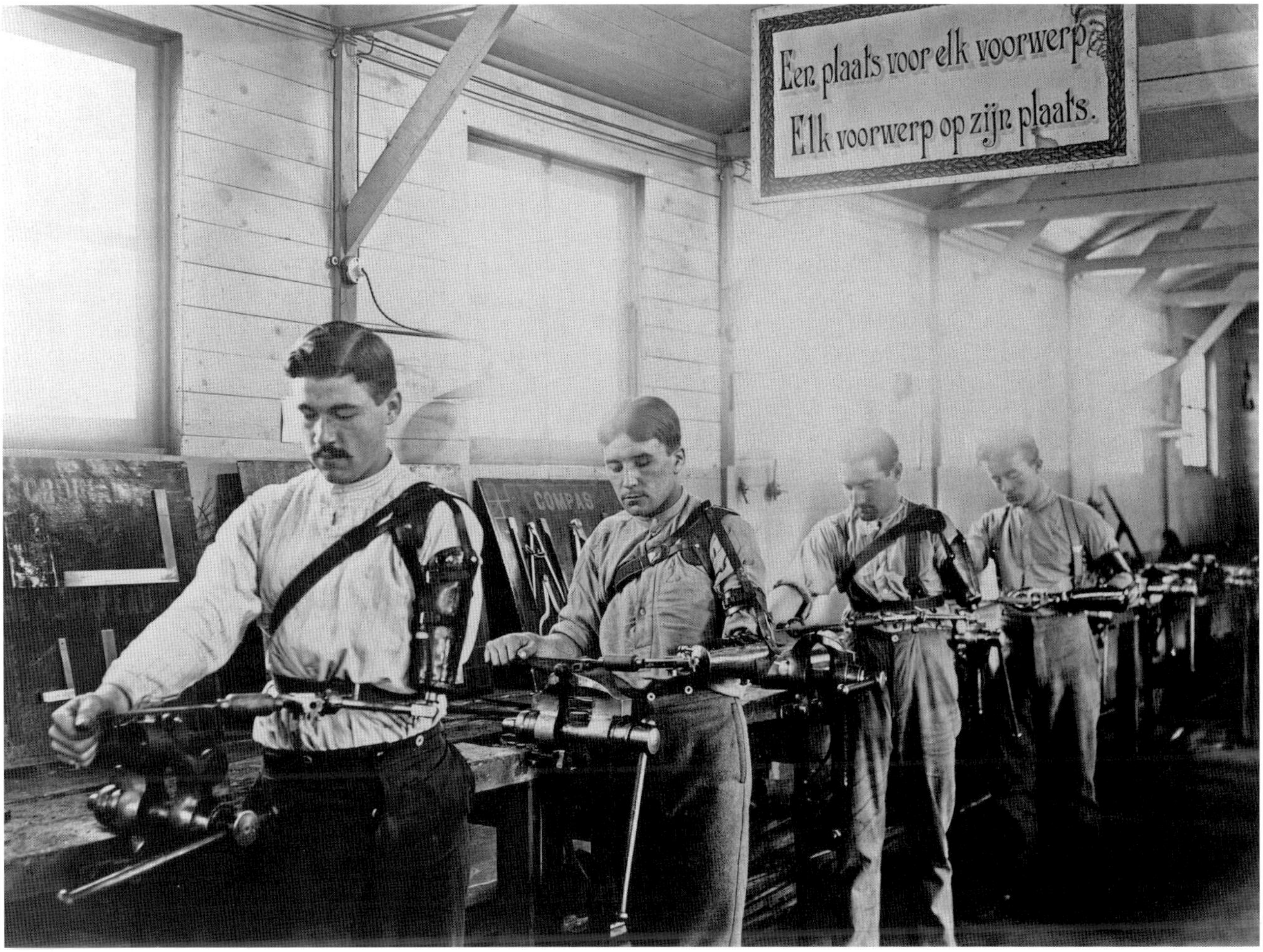
Een plaats voor elk voorwerp
Elk voorwerp op zijn plaats.
COMPAS

plaster cast, healed because they had been packed with gauze-impregnated sulpha before casts were applied. This healing process was accelerated in desert warfare because of the presence of maggots in wounds. The Trueta method was adopted by the British and US armed forces during the Second World War and by NATO forces in Korea. The introduction of penicillin and improvements in resuscitation and radiography also prompted new orthopaedic techniques. Internal nail and wire fixations were used for fractured bones and laminectomies were performed on soldiers with cervical spine injuries to decompress their spinal cords. Cervical spine injuries were also common in aircrew, and subsequently fighter pilots continued to suffer with neck and back pain caused by seating position, restricted movement in cockpits and the effects of G-force on their bodies. This was compounded by the need to wear night-vision goggles and equipment-loaded helmets. Extensive research efforts were initiated by the RAF to mitigate against these problems, such as an assessment of pilot limitations of sitting eye height in a multi-role combat aircraft. Research programmes also examined effective fields of internal cockpit vision and addressed the need to improve equipment. New exercises were introduced to strengthen pilots' neck muscles, but they continued to develop cervical osteocytes.[1]

Nevertheless, there were ongoing orthopaedic successes. Amputation rates were lowered to 8% because of improved casualty evacuation and antibiotics, although severe winters in Korea generated an upsurge in extremity surgery for frostbite. Raul Rendon, who was awarded the Purple Heart for bravery in Korea described his experience:

> *One morning I was doing an inventory of myself. I was in a hell of a mess – wounded in both hips through and through, a burn on my belly, frostbite on both feet, nose, ears*

ABOVE Four Belgian First World War veterans with prosthetic arms working machinery in 1917. *(Shutterstock)*

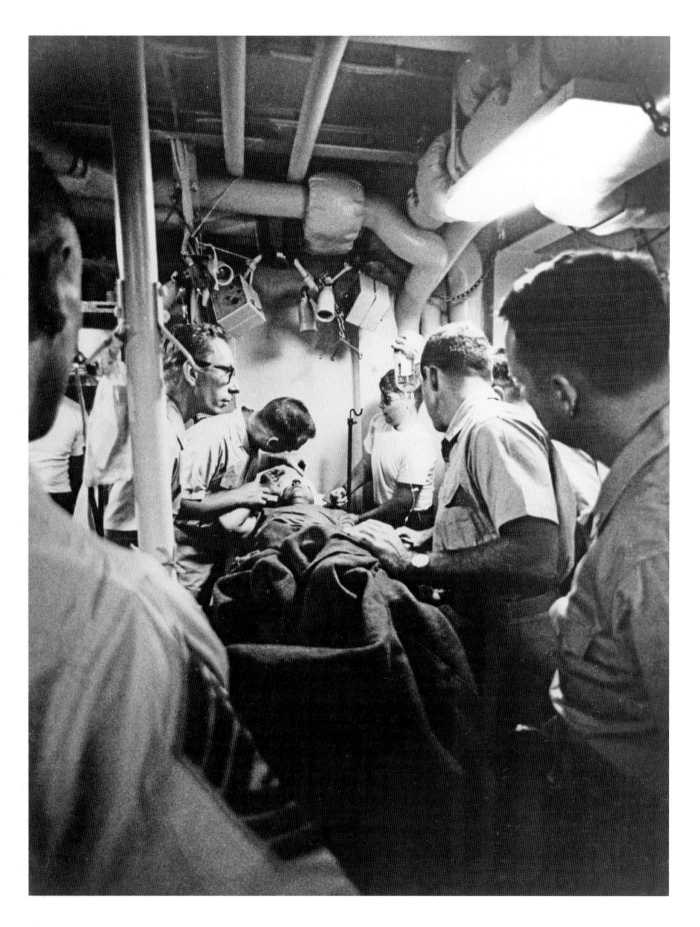

and fingers on both hands. But my feet were the worst. I was in a full body cast, both legs apart. I was given a coat hanger to scratch under my cast. I could not even clean my tail. I had tubes in me and both feet were black with frostbite and gangrene. Then I had an allergic reaction to penicillin. In Yokosuka hospital, the nurses and corpsmen called me Fred Astaire. Even though I was in a body cast, my right foot kept moving – even when I was sleeping. Because of my frostbite, I got three shots of brandy, one at each meal. But I didn't care for it, so the corpsmen asked if they could have it. I wanted candy instead. So, they got me a box of Bit-o-Honey and a box of Mars bars. The nurses always came over to see if there was anything we needed. They tried to comfort us, especially the marines like me who could not move.[2]

Frostbite injuries were measured in degrees of severity. Casualties with first-degree frostbite experienced numbness, swelling and redness of skin. Second degree produced vesiculation or perforation of the skin but affected only superficial skin layers, while third-degree frostbite penetrated the entire thickness of the skin and soft tissues. The condition usually affected the big toes, second toes, heels and fingers. Fourth-degree frostbite penetrated skin, soft tissue and bone, resulting in the need for amputation. Areas affected were treated with oxide ointments and penicillin. Anaesthetic ointment was used to relieve pain and patients were encouraged to walk as much as possible to stimulate their circulation.

Over 15% of non-battle injuries in Korea were due to the extreme cold, and over 5,000 US casualties of cold injury required evacuation

OPPOSITE US Navy doctors assess the extent of an injured Marine's wounds, October 1967.
(US Navy photo)

BELOW Hospital corpsmen bind an injured Marine's arm and chest following treatment aboard USS *Repose*, October 1967.
(US Navy photo)

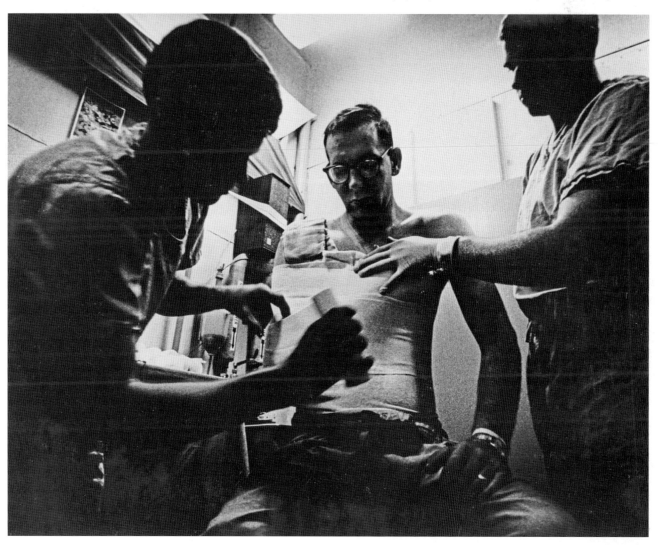

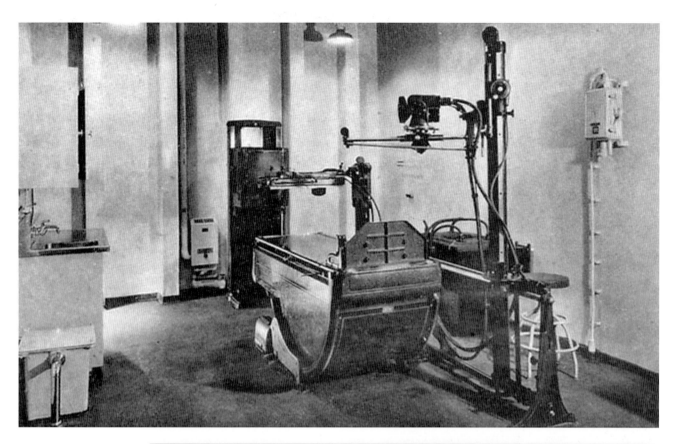

ABOVE The X-ray room aboard ship. Despite being overused during the 1950s and '60s, X-rays were an important diagnostic tool.
(US Navy photo)

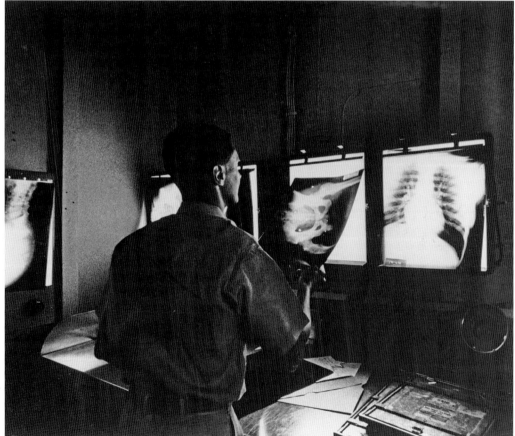

RIGHT A US Navy corpsman examines an X-ray of an injured Marine.
(US Navy photo)

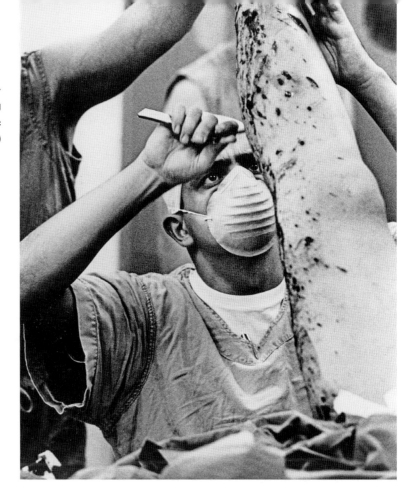

during the winter of 1950/51.[3] Most cases resulted from a combination of wet feet, immobility because of tactical considerations, inadequate body protection and sub-zero temperatures. Alcohol was prescribed to improve blood flow and was enjoyed by most patients. Staff were later instructed not to give soldiers coat hangers or other implements to scratch under their plaster casts because this practice led to a rise in infection rates. External fixations for bone injuries were also banned for the same reason. Fractures in long bones were stabilised using intra-medullary nails. In addition, physiotherapists proved their worth by manually massaging limbs, encouraging post-operative exercises and stimulating nerve pathways with electronic massage machines. They also ensured that massage, cupping and breathing exercises significantly improved patient's pulmonary function following surgery. Moreover, by treating minor muscular problems such as ankle sprains and torn ligaments, physiotherapists did much to alleviate the workload of combat surgeons and maintain the fitness of fighting units. Australian forces were among the first to deploy them in forward areas, to mitigate against back problems and other non-battle injuries.

Surgery on extremities continued to feature prominently in Vietnam where booby traps and land mines increased lower-limb injuries by 300% compared to the Second World War, and over 5,000 US troops lost limbs in Vietnam.[4]

A prevalence of enemy booby traps dramatically altered injury patterns in Vietnam. Some of the worst injuries were inflicted by sharpened bamboo sticks known as 'punji sticks'. These were hidden in forested areas and were particularly dangerous; sections

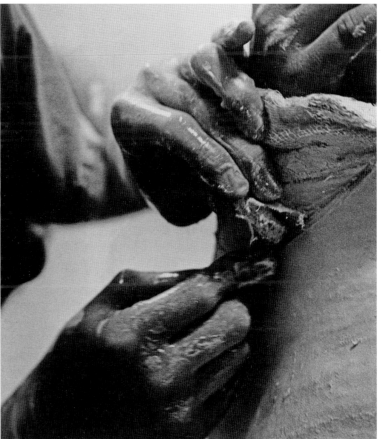

SURGICAL PROCEDURES FOR AMPUTATIONS

1 Axial skin incision (debridement) in order to decompress wound and allow post-traumatic swelling without constriction. These incisions should not cross joints longitudinally.

2 Contamination should be removed, and non-viable tissue excised. Skin is resilient and only minimal excision is necessary, typically around the margin of the wound.

3 All foreign material should be removed from wound, but obsessive pursuit of small metallic debris is not worthwhile. All dead contaminated tissue should be excised but determining the extent of tissue that should be removed is often difficult. Dead muscle is dusky in colour, shows little tendency to bleed and does not contract to forceps pressure.

4 Bone fragments denuded of soft tissue attachment should be removed. If they are left in the wound, they will become infected and form osteomyelitic sequela. Nerves or tendons should be marked with suture for future repair. At the end of the procedure wound is washed with copious amounts of saline and left open. A bulky dry sterile dressing is applied.

Source: S.J. Mennion, 'Principles of War Surgery', *British Medical Journal*, 330:1498, 23 June 2005.

BELOW Fake wound on a hand for learning in simulation training. Hand surgery gained prominence during the Vietnam War, with a greater use of delicate wires and ortho-plastic techniques. *(Shutterstock)*

of the stick could infiltrate wound tracts and cause infection deep into the bone and tissue. Since the enemy constructed these weapons by dipping 'punji sticks' into faecal matter before use, it was not surprising that wound infection rates rocketed.[5] Vietnam's hot, humid environment was a breeding ground for bacteria, with tibia and fibula fractures commonly infected. The anterior tibial region usually presented a challenge for orthopaedic

specialists because wounds were usually of an extensive nature associated with a dubious blood supply. Sepsis caused by Pseudomonas and Klebsiella was common, and despite the use of antibiotics, osteomyelitis (bone infection) was a frequent reason for lower-limb amputation.

With limb injuries accounting for over half of combat-related trauma there was a shift in clinical attitudes towards amputations. This was demonstrated by a marked reluctance to perform primary amputations, and a gradual abandonment of guillotine amputations (although still performed in an emergency) previously favoured by the military. Complex multiple injuries also fostered a relationship between orthopaedic specialists and plastic surgeons. More thought was given to achieving optimal function of the surviving stump and of retaining as much of the limb as possible. All amputations were carried out using tourniquets to stem haemorrhage and orthopaedic surgeons advocated the use of a myoplastic flap to cover transected bone.[6] Rectus abdominis and latissimus dorsi flaps had the potential to compromise rehabilitation and future mobility, which depended on truncal and upper limb strength.[7]

From Vietnam onwards, primary wound closure was delayed, to allow time for swelling to subside and any infection treated. Head and facial wounds were exceptions to this policy, because the abundant blood supply to the head acted as a powerful deterrent to infection.

Furthermore, advances in hand reconstruction featured strongly in Vietnam, performed by surgeons who had a combination of orthopaedic knowledge, neurological dexterity and plastic surgery skills. With a high incidence of lower-leg amputations among combat wounded, it was considered a priority to save hand function for rehabilitation purposes, since the hands of amputee patients would be needed to propel wheelchairs and fix external prosthetics. Severe hand injuries in Vietnam were successfully treated by initial

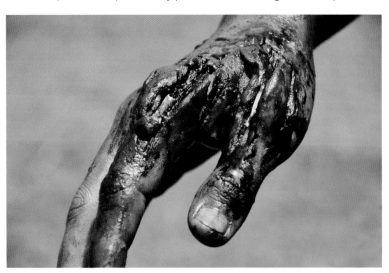

OPPOSITE Navy surgeons perform surgery on a wounded Marine aboard USS *Repose*, October 1967. *(US Navy photo)*

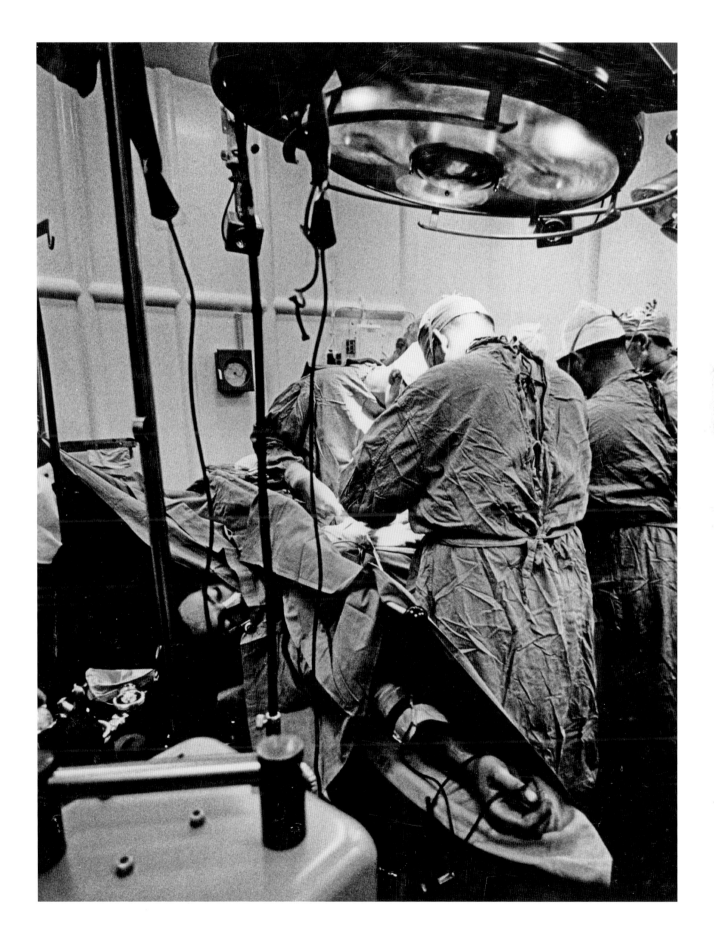

operations to assess and clean wounds, followed by secondary operations a few days later, to repair nerve, bone and tendon damage. Kirschner wires were sometimes inserted to fix small bones together. These were later removed once healing had taken place. In later conflicts members of orthoplastic teams were able to take advantage of new radiographic imaging such as image intensifiers and scans, which magnified nerves, small blood vessels and tendons, to facilitate accuracy in surgical approaches. Orthoplastic surgeons also stressed that all wounds needed to be examined outside the zone of injury to avoid accidental damage to neurovascular structures in disrupted anatomy and to allow comparison between barely damaged, vulnerable but viable and necrotic tissue. They also noted that topical negative dressings (TND) were shown to be very effective for dressing ballistic wounds. These dressings removed exudate and improved blood flow to wounds.[8]

Field hospitals, however, were often basic, and during the Falklands Campaign

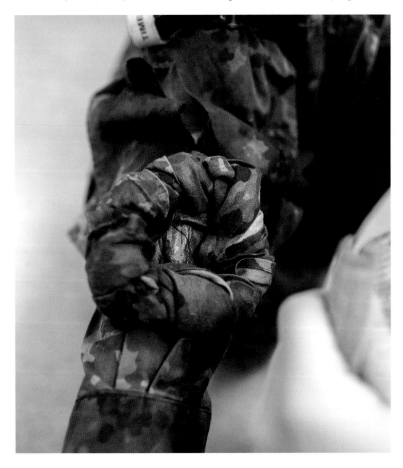

orthopaedic surgeons did the best they could without X-ray equipment.

To the modern surgeon the idea of operating on broken bones and wounds with foreign bodies without the aid of radiographs may seem tantamount to negligence, but the experienced war surgeon relies on his eyes to explore a wound that he has already made large enough for the purpose. It was interesting to note that although operations in the field were carried out without gowns (but with gloves and an apron) masks were worn. Most of the wounds were of the limbs but penetrating wounds of the skull, the chest and the abdomen were dealt with successfully in primitive conditions.[9]

Thomas splints were not used in the field because of the cumbersome shape of the splint, and the weight this equipment would add to the 60kg soldiers were already required to carry. Splints were available on the troopship *Canberra* and on the hospital ship *Uganda*, but some 'soldiers' thighs were so well muscled that even the largest rings had to be cut'.[10]

By the 1990s new orthopaedic implants and prosthetics were devised that were lighter and more flexible. But during Operation Freedom and Operation Enduring Freedom the range of injuries caused by mortar fire, grenades and the newly emerging IEDs became more severe. The extremely high pressure caused by one or more detonations of an IED created blast winds, otherwise known as 'shock fronts'. While protective clothing and helmets lowered deaths from gunshot wounds to under 5% during the Iraq wars, musculoskeletal injuries accounted for over half the wounds and presented orthopaedic surgeons with a new, multiple and complex set of problems: mangled limbs, catastrophic haemorrhage, breathing difficulties, vital organ damage, an array of compound fractures, burns, facial and sensory injuries. Casualties from IEDs were barely recognisable as human beings, their whole bodies shattered and ripped violently open as blast shockwaves inflicted a lethal combination of sharp, penetrating wounds, and multiple organ failure.[11] To an extent some medics were more prepared to care for such dreadful injuries than

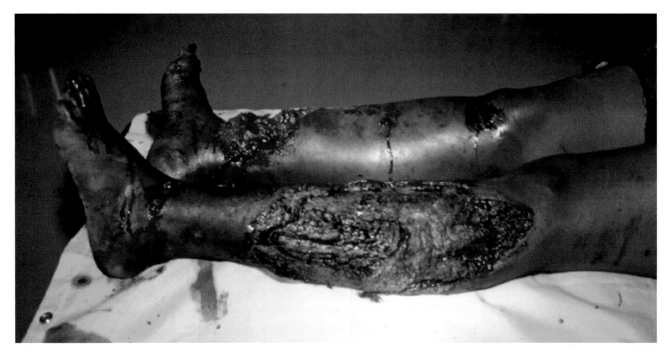

ABOVE Mangled legs: blast injury before wound excision (top) and after wound excision (bottom). *(Crown Copyright Open Government Licence)*

BELOW Lower leg trauma due to blast injury. *(Crown Copyright Open Government Licence)*

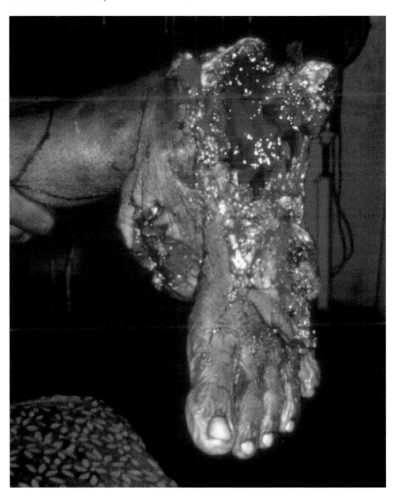

CATEGORISATION OF BLAST INJURY

1. Primary blast injury: is experienced by casualties close to explosion and is due to interaction of this shock front on air-filled cavities within the body, such as the middle ear, lung and bowel.

2. Secondary blast injury: is due to impact on body in terms of energised explosion. Modern munitions contain pre-formed metallic fragments, lacking aerodynamic features, such fragments rapidly lose velocity, which results in low energy transfer pattern wounds.

3. Tertiary blast injury: is seen when victim is accelerated by the blast and thrown against a fixed object such as a wall.

4. Quaternary blast injury: is caused by the collapse of any building secondary to a blast event.

Source: S.J. Mennion, 'Principles of War Surgery', *British Medical Journal*, 330:1498, 23 June 2005.

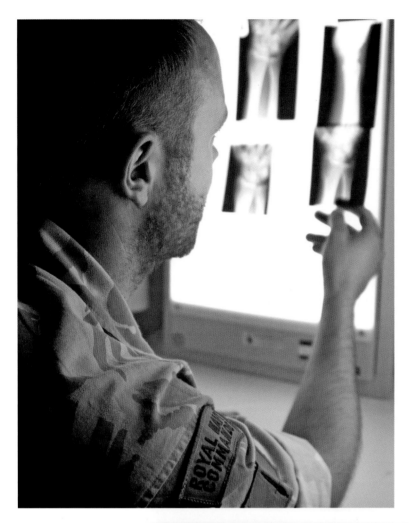

they had been in previous conflicts – simulated pre-deployment Multiple Amputation Trauma Training (MATT), using animatronics and state-of-the-art technology, provided the essential groundwork for confronting trauma injuries. Medical care was also given to Iraqi and Afghan civilians, some of whom sustained injuries as a result of enemy action.

Survivors of IED blasts received appalling injuries, all of them requiring the skill of orthopaedic surgeons. Mortar attacks could also prove fatal. Dr Atul Gawande, who served in Iraq and Afghanistan with US and coalition forces, acknowledged that those injured in these conflicts represented the largest burden of casualties the US military has had to cope with since Vietnam. He described a young airman with multiple injuries:

In extremis from bilateral thigh injuries, abdominal wounds, shrapnel in the right hand, and facial injuries he was taken from the field to the nearby 31st combat support hospital in Balad. Bleeding was controlled, volume resuscitation begun, a guillotine operation at the thigh performed. He underwent a laparotomy with a diverting colostomy. His abdomen was left open, with a clear plastic bag as covering. He was then

ABOVE A Royal Navy Commando radiologist examines an X-ray at the Camp Bastion Medical Facility, Afghanistan. *(MOD Open Government Licence)*

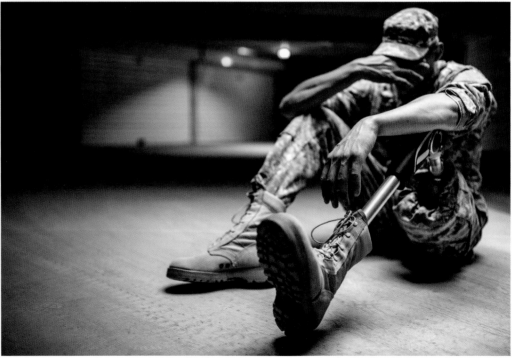

RIGHT A young amputee soldier, alone inside a bunker, cries after dealing with great trauma. *(Getty Images)*

taken to Landstuhl by an Air Force Critical Care Transport team. When he arrived in Germany, Army surgeons determined that he would require more than 30 days' recovery, if he made it at all. Therefore, although resuscitation was continued, and a further washout performed, he was sent on to Walter Reed. There, after weeks in intensive care and multiple operations, he did survive. This is itself remarkable. Injuries like his were un-survivable in previous wars. The cost, however, can be high. The airman lost one leg above the knee, the other in a hip disarticulation, his right hand, and part of his face. How he and others like him will be able to live and function remains open to question.[12]

One of the major problems confronting amputees was the level of pain experienced post-operatively; both in the short and long term. Phantom limb (still feeling pain in the limb which is no longer attached to the body) was common initially and in some patients took weeks or months to subside. Residual limb pain remained a problem for over 75% of amputees, along with associated back pain. Patients also felt joint pain in remaining intact limbs. Taking care of the stump area was

another ongoing concern, primarily to keep it infection free and fit for prosthetic attachment. Furthermore, over 60% of amputees experienced a condition known as heterotopic ossification (where abnormal bone growth exists in soft tissue areas).

As a result of experience gained in numerous conflicts, orthopaedic and orthoplastic surgery and treatment evolved to deal with more complex injuries on the battlefield. Indeed, orthopaedics and trauma care were inextricably linked. There were at least five orthopaedic surgeons in forward CSHs in Iraq, usually working alongside general and specialist surgeons. When service personnel were severely injured, often in austere combat zones, events spiralled out of control, instantaneously and unpredictably. In these circumstances access to rapid first aid and pre-hospital care was essential. First response medics launched into action to prevent catastrophic bleeding, maintain airways and breathing, stabilise fractured anatomical structures and prevent organ spillage. Once injured personnel arrived at a military care facility, resuscitation, begun at the point of injury, was a continuous process; following the <C> ABC protocol of controlling catastrophic bleeding, maintaining airway/ breathing and improving circulation.

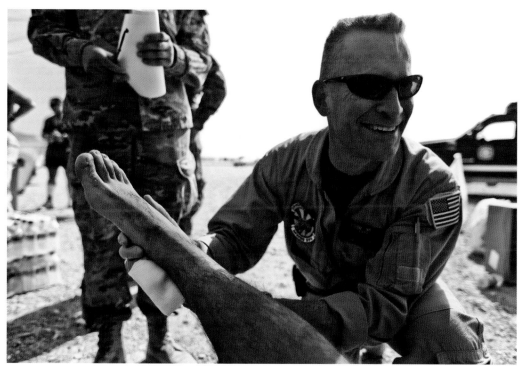

LEFT US Navy Commander Daniel Holman treats a Marine with a foot injury sustained during the Marine Corps Marathon Forward at Camp Leatherneck, Afghanistan, on 30 October 2011. *(US Department of Defense)*

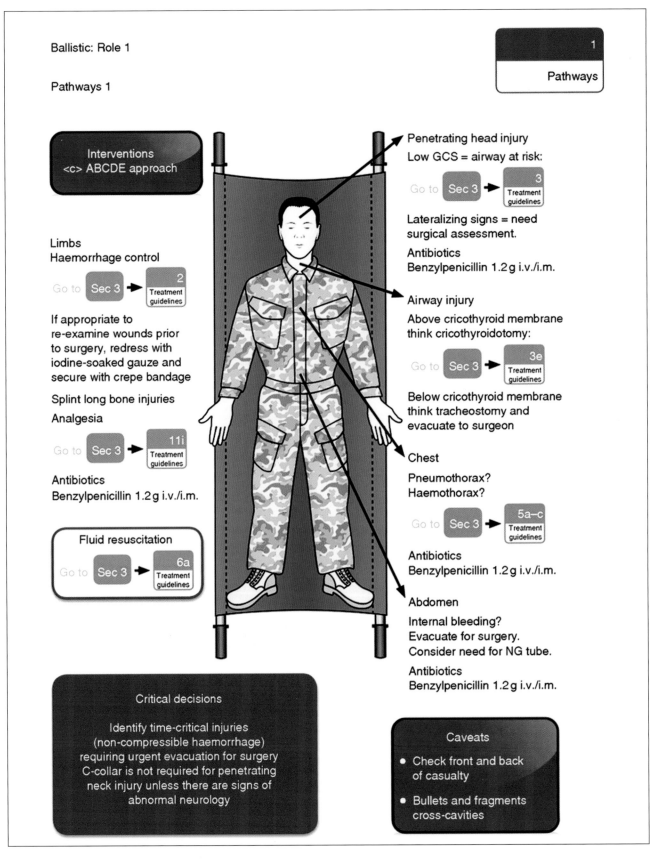

Interventions
<c> ABCDE approach

Limbs
Haemorrhage control

Go to Sec 3 → 2 Treatment guidelines

If appropriate to re-examine wounds prior to surgery, redress with iodine-soaked gauze and secure with crepe bandage

Splint long bone injuries
Analgesia

Go to Sec 3 → 11i Treatment guidelines

Antibiotics
Benzylpenicillin 1.2 g i.v./i.m.

Fluid resuscitation

Go to Sec 3 → 6a Treatment guidelines

Penetrating head injury
Low GCS = airway at risk:

Go to Sec 3 → 3 Treatment guidelines

Lateralizing signs = need surgical assessment.

Antibiotics
Benzylpenicillin 1.2 g i.v./i.m.

Airway injury
Above cricothyroid membrane think cricothyroidotomy:

Go to Sec 3 → 3e Treatment guidelines

Below cricothyroid membrane think tracheostomy and evacuate to surgeon

Chest
Pneumothorax?
Haemothorax?

Go to Sec 3 → 5a–c Treatment guidelines

Antibiotics
Benzylpenicillin 1.2 g i.v./i.m.

Abdomen
Internal bleeding?
Evacuate for surgery.
Consider need for NG tube.

Antibiotics
Benzylpenicillin 1.2 g i.v./i.m.

Critical decisions

Identify time-critical injuries (non-compressible haemorrhage) requiring urgent evacuation for surgery C-collar is not required for penetrating neck injury unless there are signs of abnormal neurology

Caveats

• Check front and back of casualty

• Bullets and fragments cross-cavities

Ballistic trauma pathways.

Ballistic: Roles 2 and 3

Pathways 1 (Cont'd)

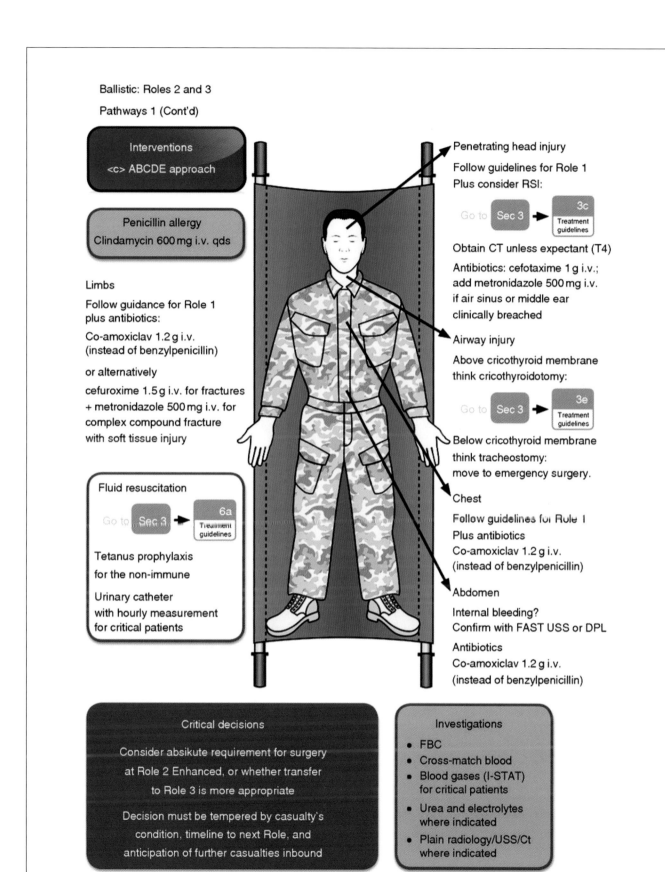

Interventions

<c> ABCDE approach

Penicillin allergy
Clindamycin 600 mg i.v. qds

Limbs

Follow guidance for Role 1
plus antibiotics:

Co-amoxiclav 1.2 g i.v.
(instead of benzylpenicillin)

or alternatively

cefuroxime 1.5 g i.v. for fractures
+ metronidazole 500 mg i.v. for
complex compound fracture
with soft tissue injury

Fluid resuscitation

Go to Sec 3 → 6a Treatment guidelines

Tetanus prophylaxis
for the non-immune

Urinary catheter
with hourly measurement
for critical patients

Penetrating head injury

Follow guidelines for Role 1
Plus consider RSI:

Go to Sec 3 → 3c Treatment guidelines

Obtain CT unless expectant (T4)

Antibiotics: cefotaxime 1 g i.v.;
add metronidazole 500 mg i.v.
if air sinus or middle ear
clinically breached

Airway injury

Above cricothyroid membrane
think cricothyroidotomy:

Go to Sec 3 → 3e Treatment guidelines

Below cricothyroid membrane
think tracheostomy:
move to emergency surgery.

Chest

Follow guidelines for Role 1
Plus antibiotics
Co-amoxiclav 1.2 g i.v.
(instead of benzylpenicillin)

Abdomen

Internal bleeding?
Confirm with FAST USS or DPL

Antibiotics
Co-amoxiclav 1.2 g i.v.
(instead of benzylpenicillin)

Critical decisions

Consider absikute requirement for surgery
at Role 2 Enhanced, or whether transfer
to Role 3 is more appropriate

Decision must be tempered by casualty's
condition, timeline to next Role, and
anticipation of further casualties inbound

Investigations

- FBC
- Cross-match blood
- Blood gases (I-STAT)
  for critical patients
- Urea and electrolytes
  where indicated
- Plain radiology/USS/Ct
  where indicated

Ballistic trauma pathways.

Blast

Pathways 2

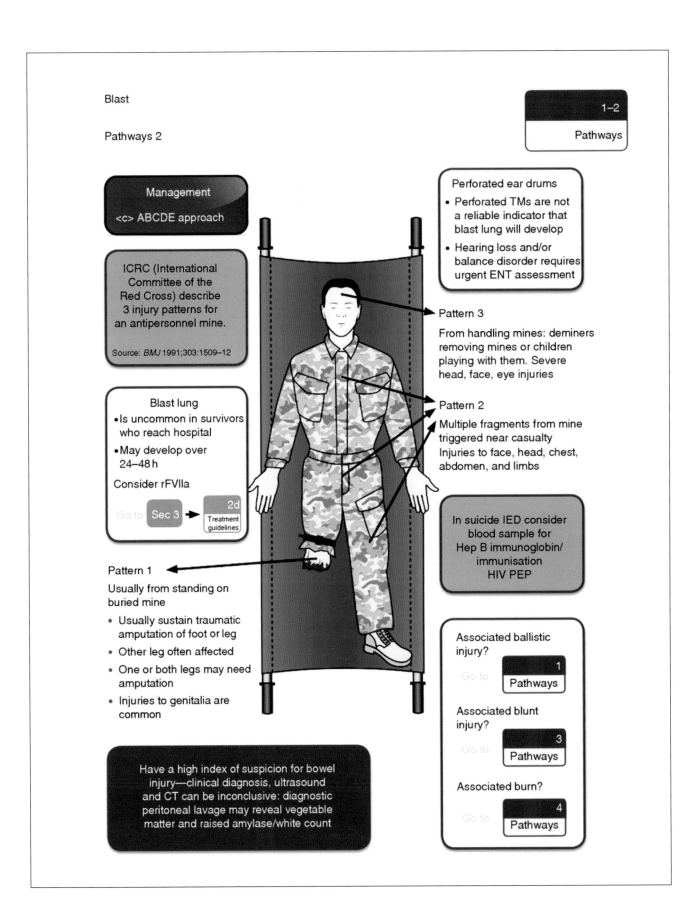

Management

<c> ABCDE approach

ICRC (International Committee of the Red Cross) describe 3 injury patterns for an antipersonnel mine.

Source: BMJ 1991;303:1509–12

Blast lung
- Is uncommon in survivors who reach hospital
- May develop over 24–48 h

Consider rFVIIa

Go to Sec 3 → 2d Treatment guidelines

Pattern 1

Usually from standing on buried mine

- Usually sustain traumatic amputation of foot or leg
- Other leg often affected
- One or both legs may need amputation
- Injuries to genitalia are common

Have a high index of suspicion for bowel injury—clinical diagnosis, ultrasound and CT can be inconclusive: diagnostic peritoneal lavage may reveal vegetable matter and raised amylase/white count

Perforated ear drums
- Perforated TMs are not a reliable indicator that blast lung will develop
- Hearing loss and/or balance disorder requires urgent ENT assessment

Pattern 3

From handling mines: deminers removing mines or children playing with them. Severe head, face, eye injuries

Pattern 2

Multiple fragments from mine triggered near casualty Injuries to face, head, chest, abdomen, and limbs

In suicide IED consider blood sample for Hep B immunoglobin/ immunisation HIV PEP

Associated ballistic injury?

Go to 1 Pathways

Associated blunt injury?

Go to 3 Pathways

Associated burn?

Go to 4 Pathways

Blast trauma pathways.

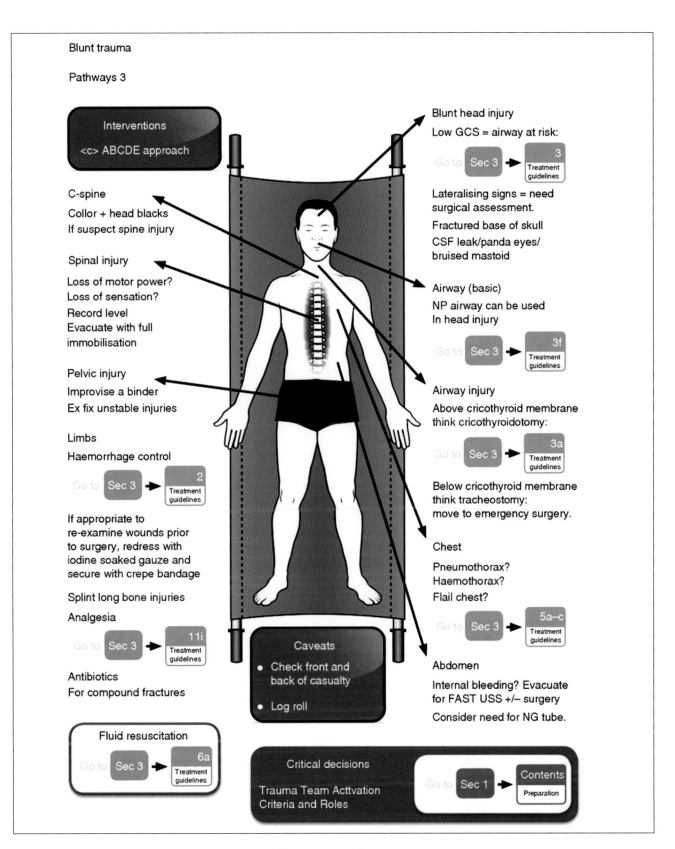

Blunt trauma

Pathways 3

Interventions

<c> ABCDE approach

C-spine

Collor + head blacks
If suspect spine injury

Spinal injury

Loss of motor power?
Loss of sensation?
Record level
Evacuate with full
immobilisation

Pelvic injury

Improvise a binder
Ex fix unstable injuries

Limbs

Haemorrhage control

Go to Sec 3 → 2 Treatment guidelines

If appropriate to
re-examine wounds prior
to surgery, redress with
iodine soaked gauze and
secure with crepe bandage

Splint long bone injuries

Analgesia

Go to Sec 3 → 11i Treatment guidelines

Antibiotics
For compound fractures

Fluid resuscitation

Go to Sec 3 → 6a Treatment guidelines

Caveats

- Check front and back of casualty
- Log roll

Critical decisions

Go to Sec 1 → Contents Preparation

Trauma Team Acttvation
Criteria and Roles

Blunt head injury

Low GCS = airway at risk:

Go to Sec 3 → 3 Treatment guidelines

Lateralising signs = need
surgical assessment.

Fractured base of skull

CSF leak/panda eyes/
bruised mastoid

Airway (basic)

NP airway can be used
In head injury

Go to Sec 3 → 3f Treatment guidelines

Airway injury

Above cricothyroid membrane
think cricothyroidotomy:

Go to Sec 3 → 3a Treatment guidelines

Below cricothyroid membrane
think tracheostomy:
move to emergency surgery.

Chest

Pneumothorax?
Haemothorax?
Flail chest?

Go to Sec 3 → 5a–c Treatment guidelines

Abdomen

Internal bleeding? Evacuate
for FAST USS +/– surgery

Consider need for NG tube.

Blunt trauma pathways.

All four diagrams highlight the critical decision-making process conducted in **NATO** Role one, two and three medical treatment facilities as casualties arrive from the battlefield. *(UK Ministry of Defence)*

Modern CSHs in Iraq and Afghanistan were geared up to admit, and successfully treat, a high volume of combat wounded. Most trauma casualties were assessed in emergency departments, while those needing urgent surgery were rushed directly to operating rooms. Doctors in charge of emergency departments supervised resuscitations, giving orders to medical staff as and when required. In the UK-led Bastion Role-three hospital, trauma/resuscitation bays all possessed the equipment necessary to administer oxygen and intravenous fluids, introduce endotracheal tubes and relieve tension pneumothorax. There were normally two anaesthetists for every resuscitation; one to ensure adequate airway and regulate anaesthetics and another to obtain vascular access. Monitoring equipment, to record vital signs, was usually attached to the patient by a nurse, who would also assist operating procedures. Tourniquets were removed or exchanged for pneumatic devices by orthopaedic surgeons once instructed to do so by the trauma lead. Radiologists were also an integral element within trauma resuscitation teams: reading X-ray films taken in emergency departments with digital portable X-ray machines and conducting ultrasound examinations of heart and abdomen (focused assessment with sonography in trauma examination), to provide immediate feedback regarding potential areas of haemorrhage and sources of hypotension. Further radiological examinations, such as computed tomography (CT) scans of the head and whole body as well as angiograms, were conducted once casualties were stable.[13]

A multidisciplinary approach was commonly used in operating rooms to ensure effective use of time and manpower. Hand specialists, for instance, reconstructed injured hands at the same time as orthopaedic surgeons performed amputations. Recent studies conducted at Bastion also suggested that multidisciplinary approaches reduced mortality rates.

Between 1 November 2009 and 30 September 2011, in 3,483 military trauma admissions at Bastion patient outcomes were as follows:

- Killed in action – 381
- Died of wounds – 37
- Returned to duty – 1,026
- Wounded in action – 3,102.

Patients admitted with signs of life had a died-of-wounds rate of 1.8% with an average 1.2 days in hospital. Therefore, we can deduce that a systematic multidisciplinary approach to trauma is associated with low in-hospital mortality.[14]

Damage-control orthopaedic surgery worked in much the same way as other specialities. Operative times were kept to a minimum, prioritising haemorrhage control and wound cleaning. Then musculoskeletal stabilisation was achieved using the minimum of invasive orthopaedic methods. Moreover, because 77% of all trauma casualties suffered from wounds which required orthopaedic intervention, this specialism was central to effective overall trauma management. One body of orthopaedic opinion, however, argued that damage-control orthopaedics versus definitive care was binary

MECHANISMS OF INJURY, BASTION HOSPITAL, AFGHANISTAN

- Improvised explosive device 48%.
- Gunshot wounds 29%.
- Other: including helicopter crash, mine, blunt object, crush, chemical inhalation injury, physical altercation, building collapse, animal bite, electrical injury and burn 7%.
- Motor vehicle collision 3%.
- Fall 4%.
- Mortar fire 2%.
- Rocket propelled grenade 3%.
- Grenade 2%.
- Machinery 2%.

Source: C. Creighton, et al., 'Trauma Care at a United Kingdom-Led Role Three Combat Hospital: Resuscitation Outcomes from a Multidisciplinary Approach', *Military Medicine*, 179 (11) (2014), 1258–62. Injuries sustained between 1 November 2009 and 30 September 2011. Average patient age: 24.4 years.

and outmoded, suggesting instead, that early appropriate care (EAC) – with its deeper understanding of trauma physiology – was a better, more fluid, approach.[15]

Appropriate orthoplastic care was crucial for subsequent rehabilitation. Indeed, a growing trend within orthopaedic surgery, to save as much limb function as possible in cases needing amputation, combined with technological advances in neuroscience and bio-engineering, has raised new hopes for the rehabilitation of amputees. United by a quest for more user-friendly multifunctional prosthetic devices, scientists have formulated innovative ways for controlling artificial limbs. Research has focused on two distinct areas of prosthetic development: in one area efforts are being made to perfect existing socket-based technology, and in another work is concentrating on integrating prosthetic systems into the body.

Existing technology already allows prosthetic fingers on artificial arms to detect temperature, pressure and movement by means of small sensors. These give signals to skin covering the stump by means of electric currents. The brain then steps in and forms new neural pathways to interpret new functions. Vision machinery is fitted to prosthetic hands and it is hoped that similar equipment will be embedded into the feet of artificial legs, to guide direction and foot placement. Prosthetic legs, however, cause more problems than artificial arms. Weight bearing inflicts more stress on the skeletal system, and results in greater friction between the stump and prosthetic. Many amputees also face the prospect of hip replacements because of imbalances in gait. Advanced lower-limb prosthetics can already adjust to ground surfaces and shifts in posture, but the expense of such devices prevents widespread use. Microprocessor-controlled knees (MPKs) also give users good stability and controls gait, swing and posture by means of battery-powered programmable software. Smart socket technology, in the form of flat

BELOW Robotic arm for human prosthesis with computer-controlled movement and motorised joint articulation. *(Shutterstock)*

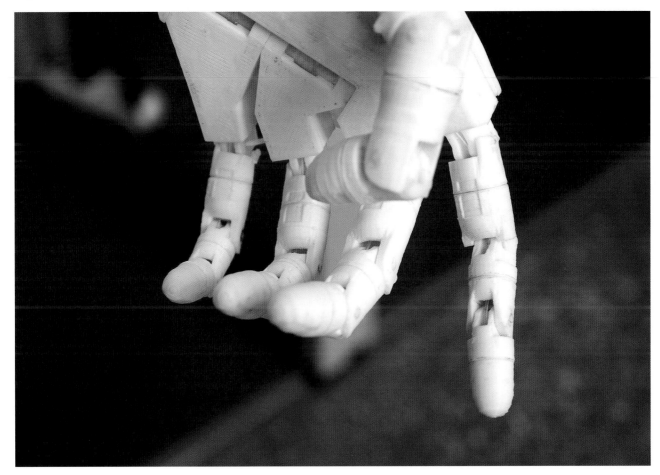

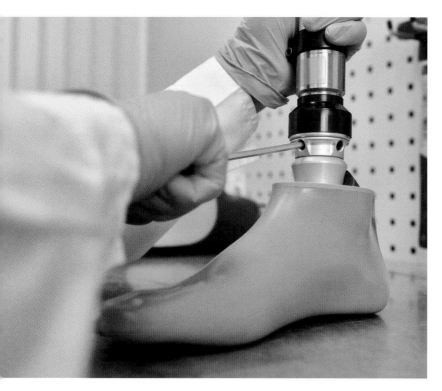

standardised interface technology which can be surgically implanted into stumps and connected to robotic limbs.

However, the real excitement in prosthetic development lies in the prospect of body-integrated systems and bio-engineering. At a fundamental level, integration involves establishing metal implant systems which can be inserted into bone shafts. Known as osseointegration, the body's natural healing capacity then forms new living bone around and within the implanted prosthetic. Advances in 3D imaging and printing are key to this process because they ensure artificial limbs are custom made, with textures that allow for the infiltration of bone. Osseointegration, however, provides a clear route for infection and ensuing osteomyelitis can risk further amputation. Therefore, softer elastomer materials designed to ensure waterproof, infection-proof seals between skin and prosthetics are being developed.

Nevertheless, the ideal is to provide amputees with robotic limbs which will feel and respond like normal body parts, and a new enterprise funded by the European Research Council aims to bring this one step closer to reality. As part of the European Union's Horizon 2020 research and innovation programme,

ABOVE A prosthetist at work on a prosthetic leg. It is the job of the prosthetist to supply artificial limbs for people who have biological limbs missing. *(Shutterstock)*

film impregnated with sensors, is also being developed; this can warn users of signs of stump infection and associated problems. This is technology which will eventually be controlled simply by downloading an appropriate app. Bio-augmentation has also created

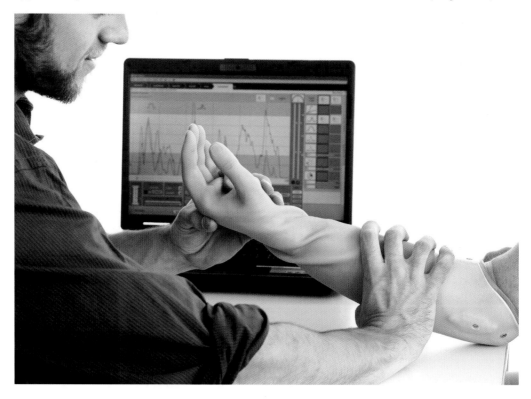

RIGHT A technician helps a patient with a prosthetic arm using a computer. The provision of artificial limbs has been greatly assisted by 3D imaging. *(Shutterstock)*

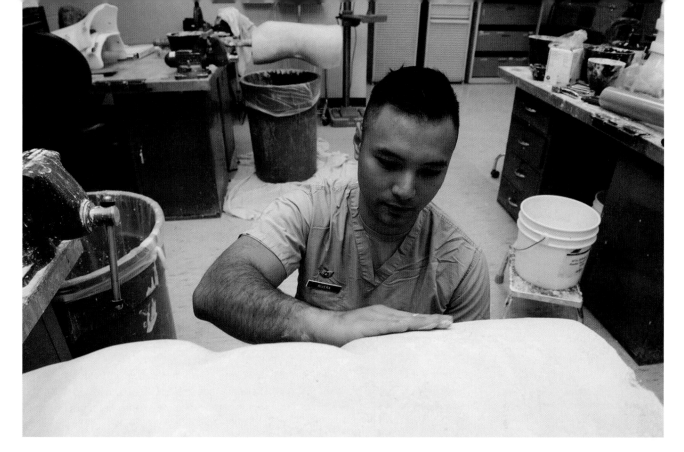

the project unites a team of scientific experts in the hope of producing bionic limbs with the ability to feel sensations and act in accordance with the user's commands. Professor Dario Farina of the bio-engineering department of Imperial College London, heads the neural interfacing team, Professor Bicchi of the Italian Institute of Technology leads research into robotics and Professor Oskar Aszmann's team, based at the University of Vienna, focuses on the neurosurgery.

Professor Farina has already produced a prosthetic hand which relies on a human–appliance interface that deciphers the user's intentions and transmits instructions to the limb. The interface has eight electrodes which receive faint electrical signals from a user's stump, which are then amplified and transmitted to a tiny computer in the prosthetic. Farina and his team intend to surgically establish a bio-hub in each amputee, in areas where nerves usually transmit control signals to missing limbs and tactile sensations to the brain are surgically directed. The bio-hub will be embedded in muscle to provide nerves for muscle movement, and in transplanted skin to establish nerves for sensitivity. As a mix of surgically reinnervated muscle and skin tissue, the bio-hub will then link to electrodes which will receive nerve electrical

ABOVE Student in orthotics. An orthotist studies for three years to obtain a BSc degree and supplies braces and splints to adults and children with a variety of spinal and limb conditions. *(US Air Force photo)*

impulses for control and sensitivity. The interfaced bio-hub will then transmit information to robotic prosthetics that mimic the natural conformity and responses of human limbs.

Speaking in October 2018, Professor Farina explained the essence of the research:

We have partly worked out how to let the brain command a prosthetic limb. Now we want to reach fully natural control and to have limbs talk back to the brain via natural sensations. Creating a hyper-reinnervated bio-hub is equivalent to building bio-connectors that will allow us to receive signals from the spinal cord and to provide sensations, such as the sense of limb position, into the spinal cord. In this way we will be able to connect the spinal cord circuitries with robotic limbs to make them a more natural part of the patient's body.[16]

This research is ongoing but has the potential to transform the lives of amputees by producing an entirely new generation of prosthetics.

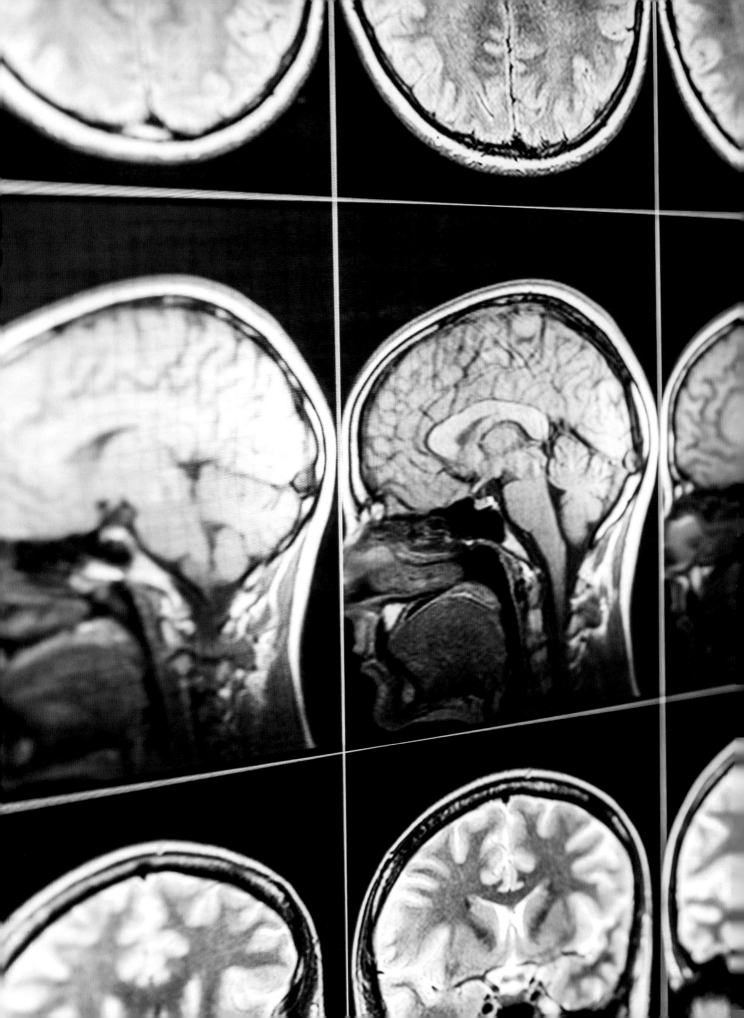

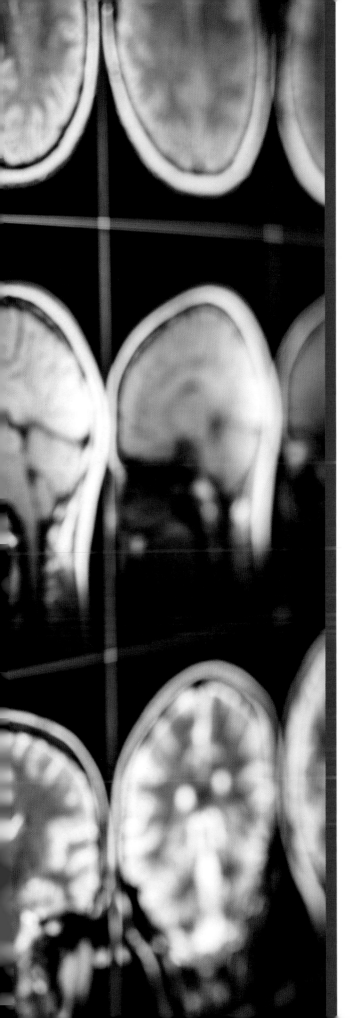

Chapter Seven

Traumatic brain and facial injuries

In the military environment traumatic brain injuries are usually caused by high-speed projectiles, gunfire or explosions. Neurosurgeons aim to preserve and restore brain function by performing surgery within 48 hours. This type of injury became known as the 'signature wound' of Afghanistan.

OPPOSITE Neuroimaging. Advances in neuroimaging have provided important information in the pathophysiology of neurological and psychiatric disorders, including the chemistry and metabolism of the brain and interconnectivity of brain cells. *(Shutterstock)*

Gunshot wounds and blast injuries have always been a feature of mechanical warfare. Propelled by kinetic energy, ballistic weapons usually cause deep, penetrating damage to bones, major nerves and blood vessels. Ballistic fractures are notoriously slow to heal, and gunshot wounds of the head require special resuscitative measures, pre-hospital care and often complex surgical interventions. Environmental conditions add to these problems, since battlefield wounds invariably contain all kinds of debris; from in-driven bone, hair and skin fragments, shrapnel shards, contaminated soil or sand and even traces of an assailant's blood or skin. Head and facial wounds are accompanied by huge blood losses and casualties often die of shock unless they receive prompt medical attention. Such injuries frequently inflict neurological trauma, damage to the cranium and underlying brain tissues, fractures of the cervical spine, damage to facial and skin structures and lesions to the eyes, ears, nose and throat. Most military traumatic head injuries are caused by high-speed projectile gunfire or explosions. In such cases military medics aim to preserve and restore brain function by performing neurosurgery within 48 hours.

BELOW Soldier with a head wound suffered during the fighting at Verdun in the First World War. *(Wellcome Collection CC-BY)*

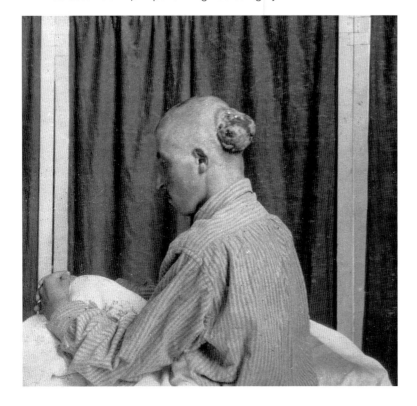

The foundations of neurological war surgery can be traced to experiments conducted by American neurologist Dr Harvey Cushing during the First World War. Faced with mounting casualties suffering from gunshot wounds and after a series of neurological operations which had resulted in failure because it was impossible to remove numerous shards of shrapnel embedded in the brain, Cushing decided that a magnet might resolve the problem. In his meticulously detailed journal, he described the first successful operation to retrieve shrapnel from the brain using a nail and magnet:

Several unsuccessful trials this morning to extract shell fragment by aid of magnet from the brain of poor Lafourcode. We had tried every possible thing in our own cabinet and in those of lower floors without success. Finally, while I was at lunch, Boothby hit upon precisely what was needed in the shape of a large wire nail about 6 inches long, the point of which he had carefully rounded off.

Well, there was the usual crowd in the X-ray room and approaching corridor, and much excitement when we let the nail slide by gravity into the central mechanism of smiling Lafourcode; for at no time did he have any pressure symptoms, and all these procedures were of course without anaesthetic. While the X-ray plate was being developed to see whether the nail and missile were in contact, who should drop by but Albert Kocher with a friend from Berne; and then shortly a card was sent in by Tom Perry's friend Salomon Reinach, Membre de l'Institut, author of the History of Religions *and much else.*

So altogether we traipsed into the first-floor operation room, where Cutler mightily brings up the magnet, and slowly we extract the nail – and then – there was nothing on it! Suppressed sighs and groans. I tried again very carefully – with the same result. More sighs and people began to go out. A third time – nothing. By this time, I began to grumble: 'Never saw anything of this kind pulled off with such a crowd before. Hoodooed ourselves from the start. Should have had an X-ray made when the man first entered hospital.' The usual thing, as when one begins to scold his golf ball.

I had just taken off my gloves and put the nail down; but then – let's try just once more! I slipped the brutal thing again down the track, 3 and ½ inches to the base of his brain, and again Cutler gingerly swung the big magnet down and made contact. The current was switched on and as before we slowly drew out the nail – and there it was, the little fragment of rough steel hanging on to its tip! Much emotion on all sides – especially on the part of A. Kocher and Salomon Reinach, both of whom could hardly bear it.[1]

Other treatments such as thorough wound debridement and the use of antiseptic irrigation fluids resulted in the first standardised protocols for brain injury management. There was considerable debate, however, as to whether wounds to the brain should be left partially open as a tract to drain any suppuration or treated with Dakin's fluid and closed. The decision to perform primary closure of the dura during neurosurgery was also the subject of much heated discourse. Regardless of these arguments, death rates remained high primarily because of limited access to surgical facilities on the battlefield.

Consultant neurosurgeon in the British Royal Army Medical Corps, Sir Hugh Cairns, resolved this problem during the Second World War by establishing mobile neurosurgical units. Coaches and trucks were converted into operating theatres staffed by specialist medical teams, which travelled as near to the front line as possible without impeding fighting forces. This ensured that casualties requiring neurosurgery could usually be operated on within 24 hours. Cairns, who was trained by Cushing, also advocated neurosurgical clinics in all major hospitals, and introduced protective helmets for military dispatch riders. At Cairns's insistence a new neurological unit was established at St Hugh's College, Oxford, which was immediately nicknamed 'the nutcracker suite'. Furthermore, working alongside Lord Howard Florey at Oxford University, Cairns and his medical teams began to use penicillin to treat wounds caused by TBIs.

Intraventricular and intercisternal penicillin was used for obvious infection/inflammation. A dosage of 50,000 units was diluted in saline and usually administered intracranially following thorough debridement. When given in such large

BELOW Human skull bones, lateral view. *(Shutterstock)*

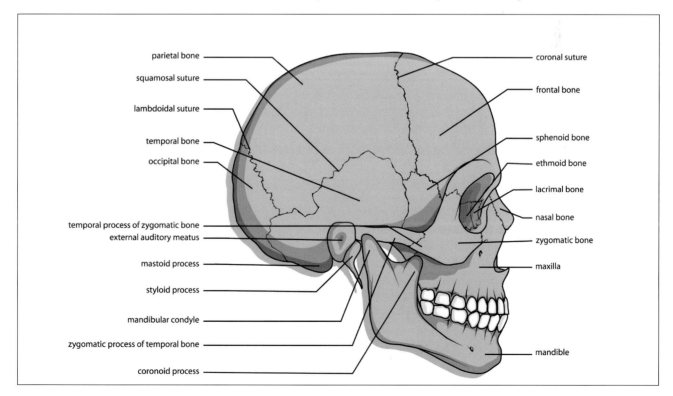

parietal bone
squamosal suture
lambdoidal suture
temporal bone
occipital bone
temporal process of zygomatic bone
external auditory meatus
mastoid process
styloid process
mandibular condyle
zygomatic process of temporal bone
coronoid process

coronal suture
frontal bone
sphenoid bone
ethmoid bone
lacrimal bone
nasal bone
zygomatic bone
maxilla

mandible

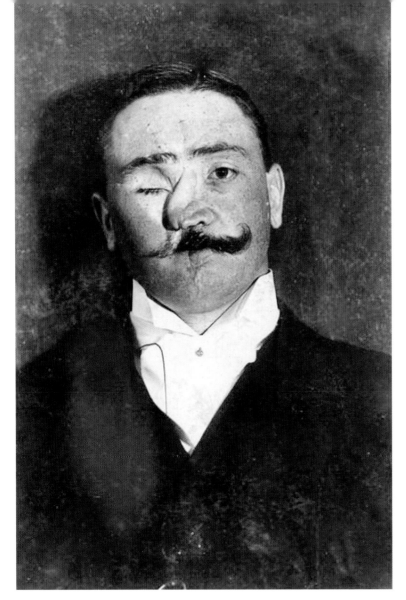

pioneering dental surgeons, and ear, nose and throat specialists. New Zealand-born Dr Harold Gillies, for instance, developed soft-tissue repairs by using pedicle skin grafts which were still attached to donor sites. He established the first designated plastic surgery unit for facial injuries at the Cambridge Military Hospital in Aldershot and the world's first facial surgery hospital in Sidcup in 1917. Nevertheless, some of the patients were so disfigured they remained in hospital for the rest of their days.

The difference in immediate casualty care by 1943 was remarkable as a matron working at a field hospital near Mount Etna explained:

We had a neurosurgical and a facial-maxillary unit attached to us and the work was very interesting. The sad part was that we could only keep our patients for so short a time; all except the dangerously ill had to go on as soon as possible, to make room for others. Rows of patients were often waiting on stretchers to go out as others were coming in.[2]

Once again mobile units made a big difference to survival rates:

Our little unit nipped about and kept as close as possible so that the men, as soon as they were wounded, got treatment on the spot. We had a fantastically high record of recovery. It was a wonderful unit to work for. I was absolutely amazed at what could be done. With men whose faces had been burned off, over several operations, flesh and skin was replaced. Noses were swung down in a flap from the forehead, even being so careful as to include a tiny edge of the hair bearing skin where it would normally meet the forehead. This was turned around into this new nose to be tucked inside the nostril so that there were hairs in the nostrils.[3]

Pilots often sustained 'airman's burns' – deep penetrating burns caused by the rapid speed with which aircraft on fire hurtled to the ground. Originally these were treated with tannic acid, which caused considerable tissue damage. But in 1940 this procedure

doses intrathecally, however, some patients experienced convulsions. In terms of surgical procedures British combat medics continued to leave the dura open during the 1940s but the scalp was usually closed. Early resuscitation and evacuation, the use of antibiotics and quicker access to definitive neurosurgery significantly improved mortality rates.

Penicillin also assisted facial-maxillary surgery. During the First World War, soldiers suffering from facial injuries were expected to walk unaided to the nearest casualty clearing station and most died of shock. Many with half of their faces blown away by the force of shrapnel and artillery fire, could not see, hear, smell, eat or drink. With shattered or non-existent jawbones they frequently bled to death before they reached a medical facility of any description. Some of those lucky enough to receive first aid and hospital treatment became patients of

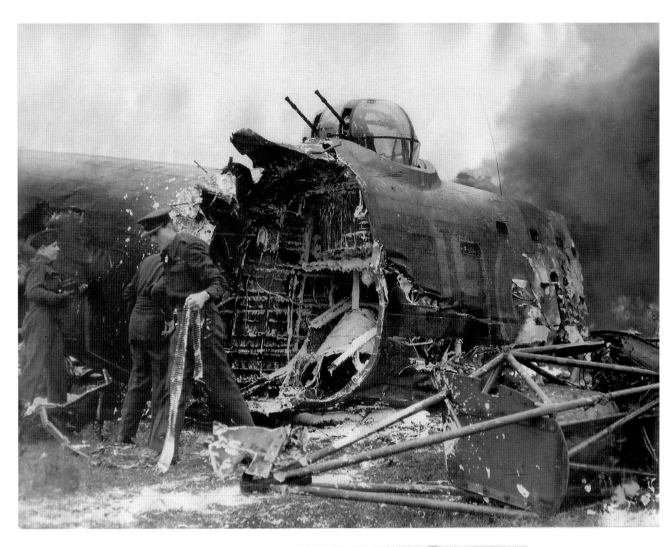

was replaced by saline infusions and 'tulle gras' dressings. Two years later the pioneering plastic surgeon Archibald McIndoe established his 'guinea pig club' at Queen Victoria Hospital in East Grinstead. Extending the principles established by his predecessor Gillies, and conducting further experimentation on the reconstruction of faces, McIndoe introduced new plastic surgery treatments. Military research scientists also began to consider ways of preventing traumatic brain and facial injuries by improving the resilience of helmets and cervical spine pads.

Clearly mobile neurological and facial-maxillary units had proved their worth during the 1940s, yet the USA was slow to implement such provision during the Korean Conflict. In the first year alone 41% of penetrating craniocerebral trauma cases developed serious infections. Delay in accessing neurosurgical

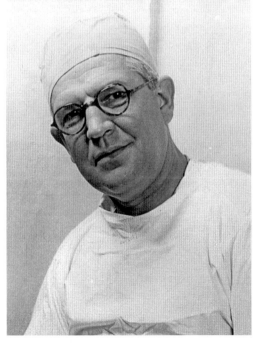

ABOVE For those airmen caught in the inferno of a crashed aircraft, the flames and extreme heat from burning metal alloys, fuel, ammunition and oxygen tanks caused terrible burns in those who were able to escape to safety. *(Jonathan Falconer collection)*

LEFT Archibald McIndoe, pioneering plastic surgeon at Queen Victoria Hospital, East Grinstead, in Sussex. *(Copyright unknown)*

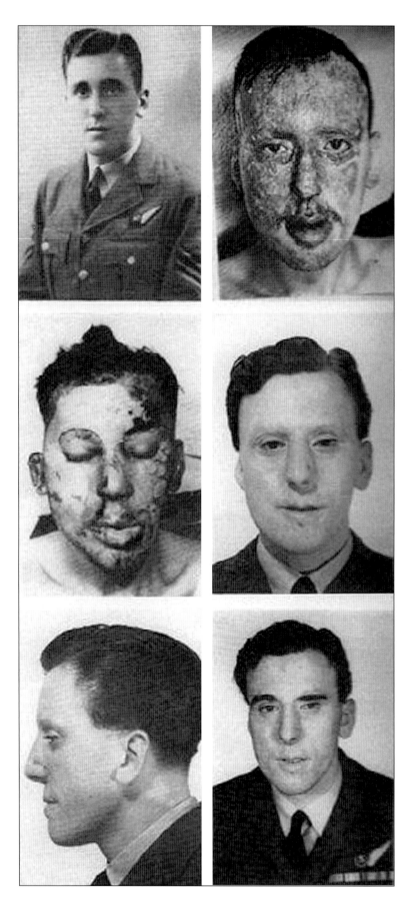

LEFT RAF wireless operator Jack Dallaway suffered extensive facial burns when his Hampden bomber was shot down by a German night-fighter intruder aircraft as it came in to land after an operation. He was one of Archibald McIndoe's patients at the Queen Victoria Hospital who became known as his 'guinea pigs'. *(Copyright unknown)*

units led to the retention of in-driven bone fragments and resultant cerebritis. This was compounded by a rise in penicillin-resistant bacteria and controversy over surgical techniques. Dural grafting and wound closure methods depended on the preference of individual neurosurgeons. Casualty care for head injuries in the early part of the war was far from ideal, and in many cases inadequate primary debridement led to fungal cerebritis, fungating fistulas and an eventual shift towards more aggressive approaches to primary wound care.

Studies of casualties from Korea, however, discovered that only half of cerebral fistulas/ sinuses were formed where bullets had entered or passed through the skull. Of these, over 70% were visible during the first two weeks of injury and 44% of this number healed without any surgical intervention. Early treatment of cerebral-spinal fluid fistulas with prompt initial resection, antibiotic-based irrigation, appropriate open wound care for hours or days and multilayered closure significantly improved patient outcomes.[4] In October 1951 US military officials recognised the growing need for front-line neurosurgeons and established the first mobile neurosurgical unit. By the following year medical care was more organised and effective. Follow-up data was also collected to determine the long-term effects of brain operations. This revealed that between 40% and 70% suffered post-traumatic epilepsy, while other neurological disorders such as aphasia and amnesia were less prominent. By 1953 watertight closure of the dura became standard practice in cases of penetrating brain trauma. This move helped to lower bacterial infection rates and lessen scar formation.

Grafts of fascia lata, other fascia such as

temporal muscle and pericranium were used in 540 successive cases. The advantages and improvement in morbidity and mortality were well documented. Infection rates declined to 1%.[5]

Brain surgery recommendations during the Vietnam War composed of total removal of bone and metal fragments, thorough and meticulous debridement, along with the practice of performing numerous operations on each patient, if deemed necessary, to prevent post-operative complications. As the war progressed, however, statistics revealed that this overly aggressive approach was detrimental to patients. Repeated operations to remove fragments in the brain increased death rates and had little or no effect on infection rates or subsequent development of epilepsy. This knowledge prompted a return to more reserved surgical approaches. Long-term head injury studies on over a thousand casualties who sustained brain injuries in Vietnam were

TRAUMATIC BRAIN SURGERY TECHNIQUE

- ■ Wound covered with sterile dressing.
- ■ Wide excision of skin edge and narrower excision of all exposed areas and periosteum.
- ■ Following close inspection, a wide excision of any exposed musculature is made.
- ■ After debridement an extension of scalp wound with a curvilinear or S-shaped incision is made using new sterile instruments.
- ■ Radius of 4cm of intact bone surrounding fracture site is exposed with removal of periosteum.
- ■ Resection of fracture site using bur holes and rongeurs as necessary.
- ■ Haemostasis and irrigation prior to opening the dura.
- ■ Excision of damaged or necrotic dural edges followed by placement of 'stay' sutures.
- ■ Cortical debridement including resection of damaged tissue and irrigation of injury track.
- ■ Most importantly, removal of clots and all bone fragments.
- ■ Removal of metal fragments if easily accessible.
- ■ Obtain haemostasis and close dura in a watertight fashion with a graft including fascia, pericranium or 'gel film'.
- ■ Close scalp with no. 0 silk sutures and cover with sterile dressing.

Source: R. Bell, C. Mossop et al., 'Early Decompressive Craniectomy for Severe Penetrating and Closed Head Injury during Wartime', *Neurosurgical Focus*, 28 (5) (2010), 1–6.

BELOW CT scan of a patient with traumatic brain injury showing a depression skull fracture in the frontal-temporal region with oedema. *(Shutterstock)*

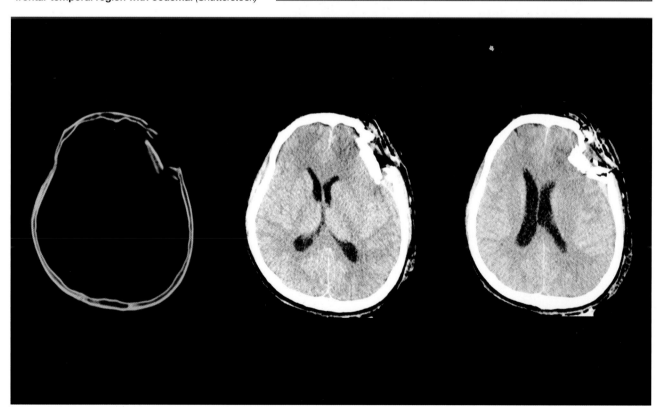

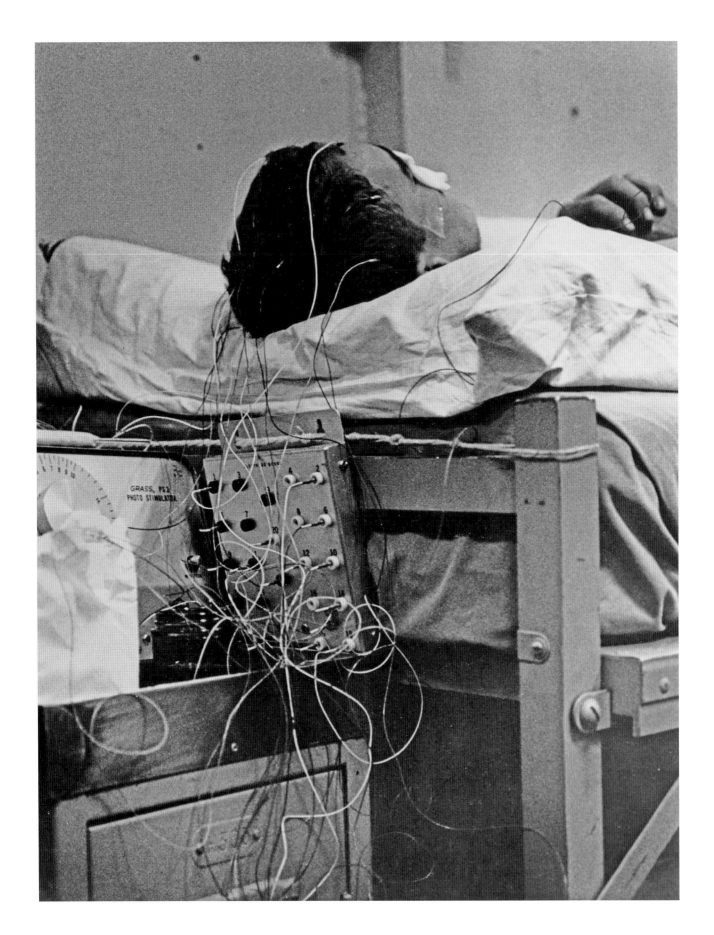

An injured man's brainwave patterns are recorded for diagnosis by electro-encephalogram (EEG), October 1967. EEGs were used for diagnosing the after-effects of traumatic brain injuries and were particularly effective at pinpointing casualties suffering from epileptic seizures. *(US Navy photo)*

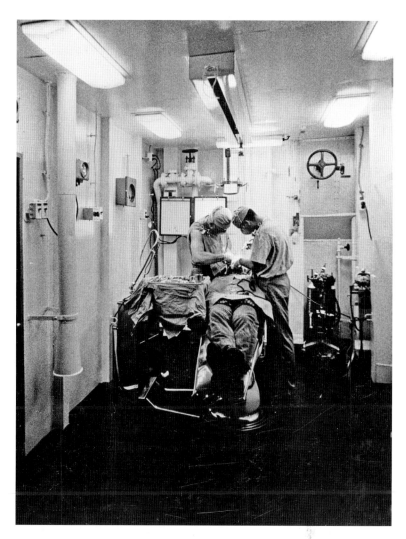

ABOVE Navy surgeons perform oral surgery, October 1967. Dental surgeons made a significant contribution to advances in maxillary/facial surgery. *(US Navy photo)*

initiated by neurologist William Caveness. These documented all cases of post-operative complications, levels of brain function, incidence of seizures, cognitive behaviour patterns, memory, dysphasia and amnesia.

In terms of facial-maxillary surgery, advances in both technique and post-operative care were features of the Korean and Vietnam wars. Fractured jaws were stabilised by using interosseous and intermaxillary steel wires, whereas mandible and mid-facial fractures were secured externally with the use of rigid frames. Orthoplastic surgery became more common and early access to surgical facilities and the systemic use of broad-spectrum antibiotics allowed for routine primary closures of facial soft-tissue wounds, along with open reduction and internal fixation techniques. Dental surgeons were deployed in forward areas and sometimes required to maintain patients' airways in the absence of an anaesthetist.

During the 1982 Falkland Islands Campaign the need for facial-maxillary surgeons and dental/oral surgeons near conflict zones was obvious. Dr Rick Jolly, Senior Medical Officer in charge of Ajax Bay field hospital, noted that the splendid Surgeon Commander George Rudge, had already 'paid his fare several times over with his expert use of the bone drill and Gigli saw to open two skulls'.[6]

Among the catalogue of horrendous injuries, burns victims accounted for 34% of casualties aboard ships during the Falklands War and 14% of overall casualty numbers. Only facial burns were left exposed, burns elsewhere on the body were treated with flamazine, intravenous fluid replacement, saline and bicarbonate, oral fluids and polyurethane foam dressings. Dr Jolly recalled 8 June 1982 when he received an urgent handwritten note from Commanding Officer John Roberts of 16th Field Ambulance, informing him of a

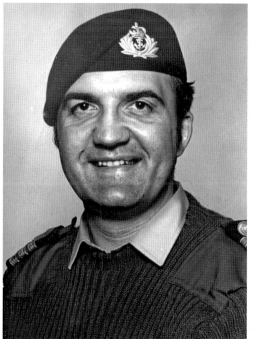

LEFT Surgeon Commander Rick Jolly, Royal Navy. *(Copyright unknown)*

mass casualty situation: 'RICK, GALAHAD HIT BEFORE SURGICAL TEAMS UNLOADED. MANY (NOT YET COUNTED) BURNS CASUALTIES NEED FLUIDS/MORPHIA PLUS PLUS – THANKS JOHN.'

Submerged in the bloody realities of war, in chaotic, pressured and challenging circumstances, Jolly and his team gradually restored a sense of order.

The fused and charred clothing was cut away, and the total percentage of burned skin area assessed and recorded on the treatment card. When necessary, an intravenous infusion was set up, with the *flow rates and volumes calculated individually depending on the burns percentage. Careful titration of intravenous morphine was then embarked on, to control the pain. Then, carefully and lovingly, flamazine was spread thickly over the affected areas. The cool white cream contained a silver and sulpha drug mixture which was pain-killing, antiseptic and promoted healing. Hands and fingers were enclosed in sterile plastic bags to avoid the risks of bandaging.*[7]

Grafting was also performed but not as a primary operation. Explosions aboard the *Sir Galahad* had caused flash burns, which lifted surface layers of skin and exposed nerve endings. These wounds were excruciatingly painful and even heavy-duty analgesics such as morphia failed to alleviate suffering. In the most severe cases ketamine was administered in addition to morphia. Escharotomies were

BELOW The Royal Fleet Auxiliary landing ship *Sir Galahad* on fire off Fitzroy after being hit in an Argentine bomb strike. Explosions and subsequent fires killed 48 men on board and wounded 97 others, and of those who survived many suffered horrific burns. *(Defence Picture Library)*

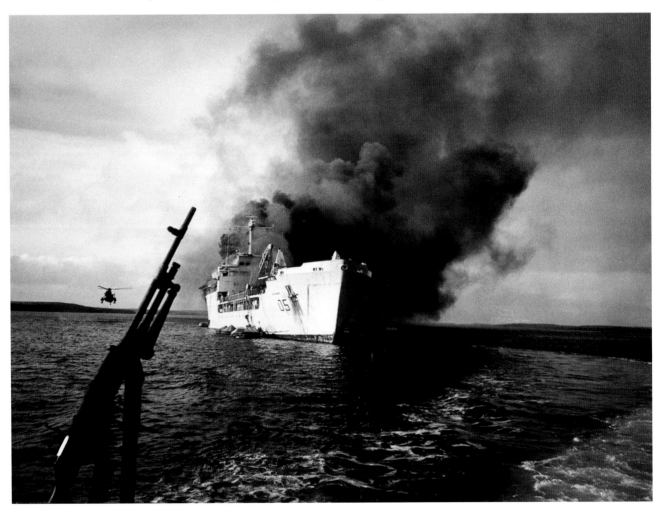

conducted on fingers to facilitate tissue fluid drainage and the effects of smoke inhalation treated with methylprednisolone. Subsequent medical reports of the Falklands Conflict highlighted the unselfish organised discipline, initiative, skill, fortitude and bravery of both combat medics and their casualties. Particularly moving was the remark of a shipwrecked rating when he learned that his captain was safe: 'If they haven't got the skipper, they haven't sunk the ship.'[8]

Advances in CT scanning techniques introduced in the mid-1980s significantly improved the outcomes of patients suffering with brain and facial wounds, not least because they revealed which patients could be treated conservatively without the need for operations. This process of elimination drastically reduced the number of patients who developed complications of brain injury, such as epilepsy. Working tirelessly in combat zones military medics remained focused on saving lives, limbs, vital organs, sight and other senses. Meanwhile, scientific research into protective combat clothing continued. Throughout the Korean and Vietnam wars the US military relied on helmets which were developed in 1941. These were designed to protect individuals from shellfire fragments rather than bullets. Fatal gunshot injuries tended to be those sustained in the occipital and frontal temporal regions – therefore, new helmets introduced in the 1980s were lighter and covered more of the head. Nevertheless, as incongruous as it may have seemed, protective headgear did not fit all head sizes. As Rick Jolly confessed of his time in the Falklands: 'I had never found a steel helmet to fit my size 8 head, so had to put my trust in the magical, shrapnel-deflecting powers of the green beret instead.'[9]

Early prototypes of face-shields, developed as an adjunct to helmets, tended to mist up or impede weapon sightings. However, more advanced personal protective clothing and equipment was developed in response to high levels of TBI in Iraq and Afghanistan. Thus, US forces wore advanced combat helmets from 2003 onwards and UK forces introduced MK 7 helmets in 2009. These models proved to be tougher and lighter, with improved fields of vision. They also offered better balance when

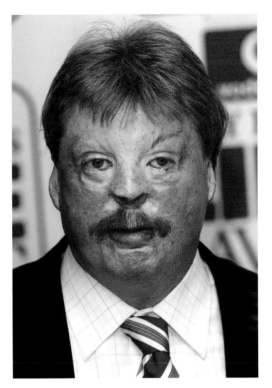

LEFT Welsh Guardsman Simon Weston, who was on board *Sir Galahad* when it was hit by an Argentine bomb, suffered 46% burns as a result of the airstrike. He underwent years of reconstructive surgery including more than 70 major operations and surgical procedures. *(Alamy)*

soldiers were required to wear night-vision glasses. Nevertheless, persuading soldiers to wear protective gear was sometimes problematic.

In Afghanistan, for instance, surgeons became increasingly alarmed by the high

BELOW Severe burns to the hand. Flash burns were problematic as they were intense and penetrated all skin layers and soft tissue. *(Shutterstock)*

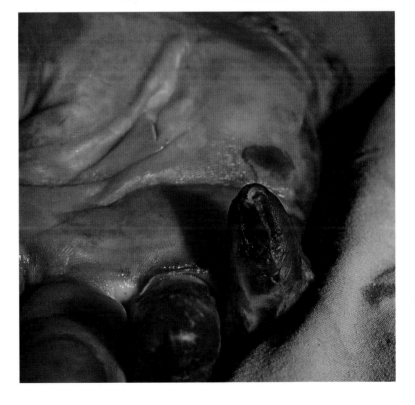

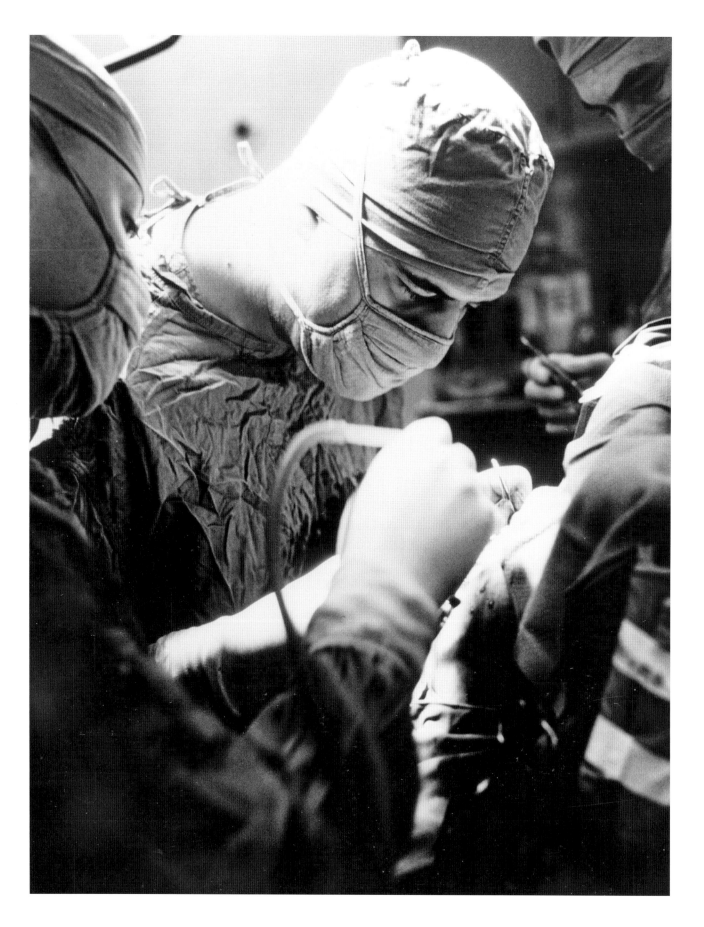

occurrence of blinding facial wounds, particularly since soldiers had been ordered to wear eye protection goggles. It seems that US soldiers had a strong sense of the aesthetic, complaining that the goggles looked like something a Florida senior citizen would wear. The military bowed to fashion and switched to cooler-looking Wiley-brand ballistic eyewear. The rate of eye injuries has since decreased markedly.[10]

The emergence of IEDs during the Iraq and Afghanistan wars dramatically increased the prevalence of TBI, to the extent that it quickly became renowned as the 'signature wound' of these conflicts. This situation prompted concerted efforts to provide more effective combat protection equipment. First-generation Head-borne Energy Analysis and Diagnostic Systems (HEADS) sensors, developed by BAE Systems, were attached to military helmets from 2007 onwards. Located under the crown suspension pads, these devices monitored combat explosions affecting the brain and over 20,000 were fitted in US Army and Marine Corps helmets. Second-generation HEADS sensors were in production by 2011. More sophisticated than their predecessors, these current devices include programmable LED lights which register explosions and indicate

KEY POINTS FOR BALLISTIC TRAUMA CONSIDERATIONS

1. Treat the patient and the wound, not the bullet or the firearm.
2. High-energy weapons can produce low-energy transfer wounds and vice versa.
3. High-energy transfer wounds evolve over several days with swelling, further tissue necrosis and exudate.
4. Ballistic fractures will be frequently slow to heal; skeletal fixation must be robust enough to protect healing fractures over the course of a delayed union.
5. Vessels distant from the permanent wound cavity may be traumatised and can represent an anastomotic risk for vascularised tissue grafting.
6. A surgeon can do more damage than a bullet with too aggressive or insufficient excision of the wound.
7. Bullets frequently ignore the rules of ballistics!

Source: Jowan Penn-Barwell, 'Ballistic Trauma Considerations for the Ortho-Plastic Surgical Team', *International Journal of Orthoplastic Surgery*, 1(2) (2018), 47–54.

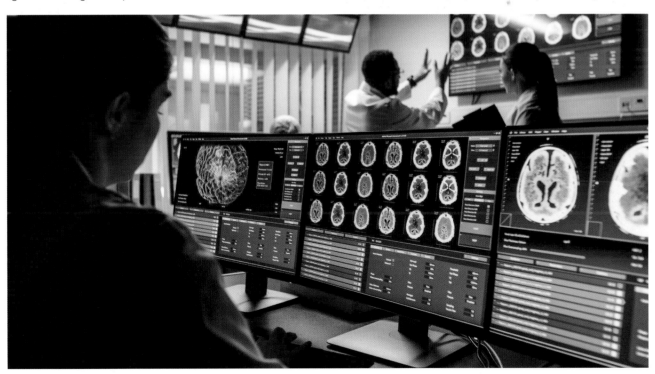

the possibility of a TBI. In addition, sensors incorporate radio frequency (RF) transmitters which are received by military personnel at a soldier's base. Other data recorded by HEADS includes the time, size, direction and extent of explosion, along with detonation pressure waves, linear and angular accelerations. This information is then downloaded for analysis by medical personnel.

Furthermore, scientists have collated TBI information depending on the method of injury: closed-head, penetrating and explosive blast TBI. They have also proposed that brain damage caused by explosive blasts is totally different to the other categories, resulting in diffuse cerebral oedema, sub-arachnoid haemorrhage, unique fractures, pseudo-aneurisms and vasospasm.[11] Moreover, the way in which detonation waves injure

the brain and central nervous system is not completely understood. Blast pressure instantly rises to above atmospheric pressure before dropping suddenly to sub-atmospheric pressure. Negative pressure may result in cavity formation in brain tissue once the blast has travelled through the skull, and/or substantial injury as the brain reacts to acceleration/deceleration pressure waves within the cranium. Furthermore, IEDs frequently caused several shockwaves as these devices tended to detonate at varying intervals. Contents of IEDs included nails, metal bolts and dirt which often resulted in a combination of blunt, penetrating and burn injuries. There were instances where victims of suicide bomb attacks even sustained wounds containing bone fragments from the assailant. Injuries from IEDs are particularly difficult to manage since they cause a wide range of blast injuries. Kevlar genital protection shields and protective vests were initially effective in terms of protecting soldiers from genital and torso injuries, but IED blasts shoot

BELOW Inspecting a bulletproof vest. Effective protective clothing is an essential component of pre-deployment preparation. *(Shutterstock)*

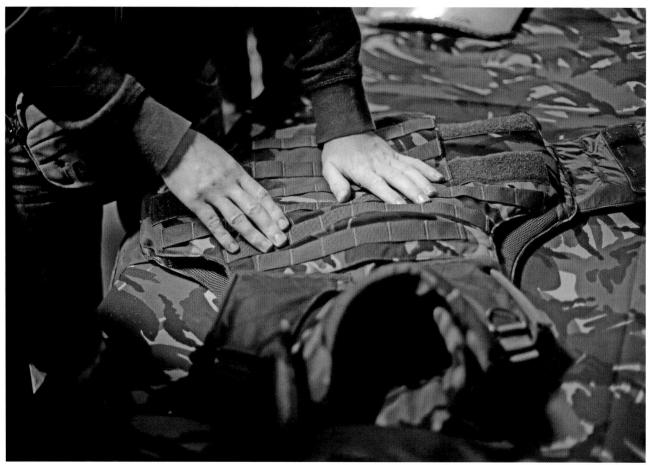

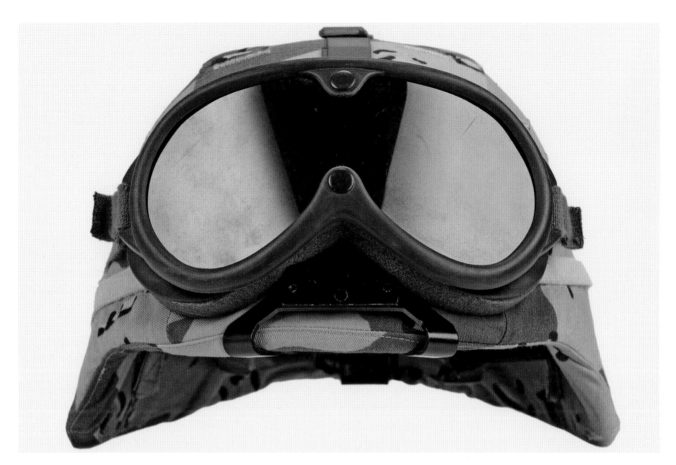

upwards under Kevlar vests and infiltrate bodies through under-arm vents. Such explosions cause multiple devastating injuries.

In trying to understand the mechanism and pathophysiology of bullet and blast injuries to the brain, scientific researchers in 2011 discovered a firm link between TBI, chronic pain and post-traumatic stress disorder (PTSD). In doing so they claimed: 'It is essential that studies recognize the close association between these areas of morbidity as markers of common pathophysiology, inter-related outcomes and therapy targets.' In other words, they shouldn't be seen or treated separately. No one should hive off psychological problems and ignore the big dent in a patient's head, the one he got from a high-velocity rifle bullet or the piece of IED. There is, in the quietly damning words of researchers, 'an entirely artificial dichotomy between neurological and psychiatric morbidity in traumatic brain injury as a whole and military traumatic brain injury in particular'.[12]

More recently scientists have discovered the presence of unique scarring patterns within the brain tissue of blast victims. Interface astroglial scarring (between white and grey matter) from blast injury samples clearly indicate that brain tissue damage worsened over time. This somewhat startling revelation heralds the prospect of new treatments for victims of brain trauma sustained as a result of military combat, particularly those suffering from PTSD, with scientists asserting that:

Our findings suggest that for the first time, there may be a predictable pattern of physical damage to the human brain after blast exposure, which standard clinical neuro-imaging techniques currently cannot detect. We anticipate reconsideration about pathophysiology underlying the neuro-psychiatric sequelae that follows blast exposure, and innovative approaches to diagnosis and treatment.[13]

Nevertheless, although these findings represent a major breakthrough in terms of understanding TBI, the process of transforming this discovery into an effective treatment for sufferers may take many years.

ABOVE Army Kevlar helmet with goggles, NVG mount and camouflage.
(Shutterstock)

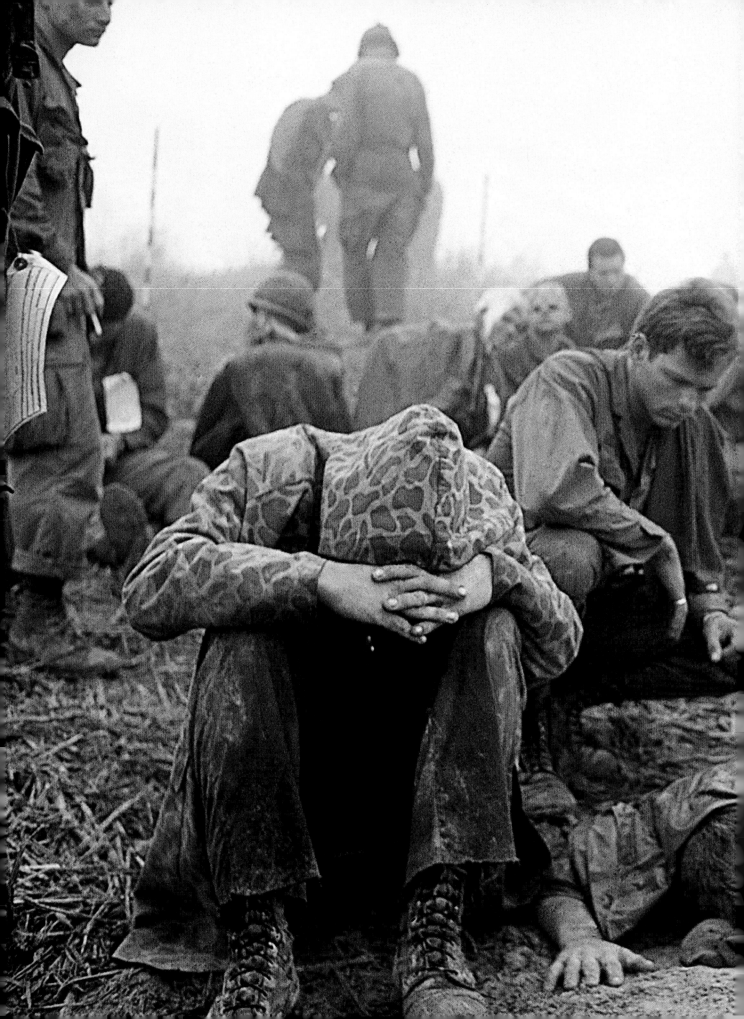

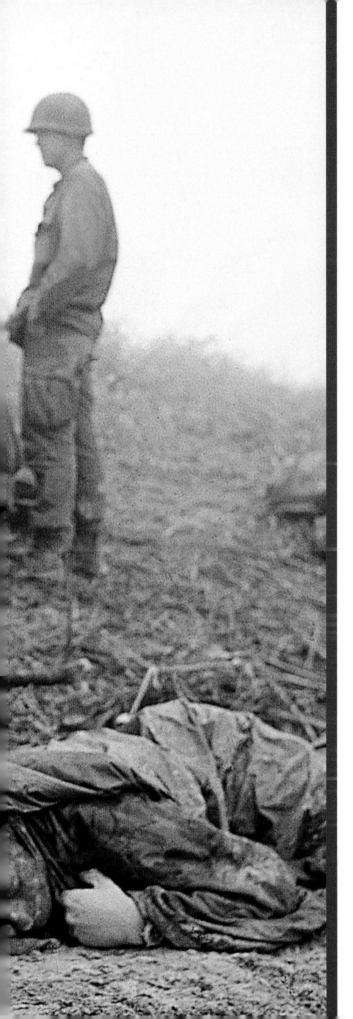

Chapter Eight

Psychological trauma

Some wounds are invisible but penetrate the mind deeper than any bullet. From shell shock to post-traumatic stress disorder the treatment of psychological trauma has been controversial. A greater appreciation of the effects of war on mental health, however, has prompted stress inoculation therapies, new medications, counselling and support networks.

OPPOSITE Wounded and traumatised soldiers from the US 1st Cavalry Division wait to be evacuated from a hilltop in South Vietnam during their advance toward Khe Sanh on 4 April 1968. *(Getty Images)*

Early recognition of psychological problems experienced as a result of combat were poorly understood, and often considered synonymous with the practice of malingering. Invisible scars of the mind, fixed in a time and place, they continued to haunt victims long after the battle was over. Between 1914 and 1916 soldiers suffering from NYDN (not yet diagnosed nervous) were pushed to far-flung corners of hospital wards and referred to as 'batty'. Growing numbers of such cases, however, prompted military alarm and a medical re-evaluation of the causes and treatment of what became known as shell shock or neurasthenia. Originally doctors believed that the condition was due to multiple minute haemorrhages in the brain, which were caused by the proximity of loud exploding artillery shells. Indeed, post-mortem examinations of men who were fatally wounded by a combination of gas attacks and artillery fire did reveal thousands of minute brain haemorrhages and initially seemed to confirm this theory. Therefore, early shell-shock victims were duly awarded a wound stripe and sent home as heroes. However, shell shock was also diagnosed in men who had never experienced artillery fire, and later

post-mortems on sufferers did not reveal brain haemorrhages. When post-mortems failed to prove a physical link between neurasthenia and loud artillery fire, attitudes towards the condition changed significantly. Suspected by many of 'swinging the lead' to avoid front-line duty, sufferers were usually ostracised by their peers and subjected to a series of medical tests designed to catch malingerers.[1]

Military perceptions of neurasthenia and its association with malingering also varied according to social class. Officers suffering from neurasthenia were rarely accused of malingering because of their elite upbringing, leadership skills and adherence to honourable principles. They were also considered to be far less likely than their subordinates to succumb to shell shock. Conversely, the presence of neurasthenia in other ranks was thought to be due to a distinct lack of moral fibre. By 1916, however, numbers of shell shock victims had substantially increased. Of those who had seen action on the Somme 40% of casualties were diagnosed with the condition and, contrary to popular military assumptions, officers were four times more likely to experience neurasthenia than the men they commanded.

Regardless of these mounting statistics, shell shock continued to be a controversial subject. A Cambridge psychologist named Dr Charles Meyers tried to prevent the execution of neurasthenia sufferers for cowardice, and to persuade senior military officials of the value of cognitive behaviour therapies. Meyers believed that sufferers could be successfully treated by rest, recuperation, talking therapies and artistic and literary pursuits. His tutor, Dr William Rivers, held similar views and established Craiglockhart military psychiatric hospital in 1916, which was nicknamed 'Dottyville' by its most notable resident, the famous war poet Siegfried Sassoon. Some 20 hospitals specialising in the treatment of shell shock were eventually established across Britain, although it was not just a British phenomenon. French and German troops also suffered from the condition in similar numbers.

Within the British military hierarchy, however, the views of Meyers and Rivers were relegated in favour of those who believed neurasthenia to be the product of emotional weakness, bouts

RIGHT **Patient suffering from war neurosis – shell shock.** *(Wellcome Collection CC-BY)*

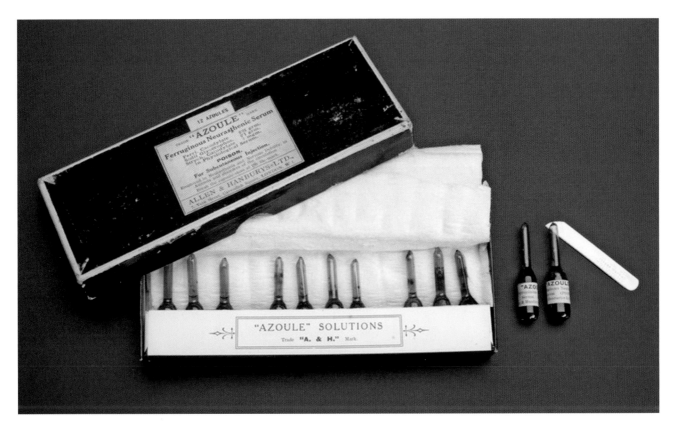

of hysteria or an excuse to escape front-line duty. Some psychiatrists refused to even accept the existence of neurasthenia. An extremely overzealous, sadistic Canadian psychiatrist named Lewis Yealland, for instance, boasted that he could return all shell-shock victims to the front line within a matter of days. He claimed to have a 100% 'cure' rate and his methods were barbaric! Uncommunicative soldiers were tied to wooden chairs while burning cigarettes were simultaneously placed on the back of their tongues and electrodes attached to their genitalia. Yealland would then administer electric shocks and loudly shout at his victims to become heroes. Soldiers were required to speak out in order to stop this torture. Those who could not were repeatedly subjected to the same treatment. For most, the horrors of the front line were infinitely preferable to the degrading and shockingly cruel tortures inflicted by Yealland and his team.

During the inter-war years, psychiatrists and psychologists helped recruitment officers in the British armed forces to devise psychometric tests for new recruits, in the hope of weeding out potential emotional weaklings. Pervading attitudes still viewed shell shock as a major

character defect and equated the condition with malingering. Thus, soldiers returning to civilian life with physical wounds were far more likely to receive favourable treatment, sympathy and respect than those who continued to struggle with mental health problems. Psychiatrists in the USA and across Europe experimented with highly controversial treatments, such as insulin therapy, electroconvulsive therapy and, in extreme cases, lobotomies. These experiments did little to change public perceptions of mental health disorders.

However, a shift in military assumptions about causes of psychiatric stress was perceptible by 1939, with the RAF taking the lead in combat stress research. Nurse Monica Baly was involved in this process:

We were investigating the stress on aircrews. We had learnt from the mistakes of the First World War, of which there were many – tragic of course. But these investigations revolutionised mental nursing. There was a changed attitude towards anxiety states, and one realised that they could be rehabilitated with counselling, psychotherapy and so forth.[2]

ABOVE Ampules of ferruginous neurasthenic serum containing strychnine cacodylate, sold as a strengthening tonic for neurasthenia, anaemia and circulation disorders. *(Wellcome Collection CC-BY)*

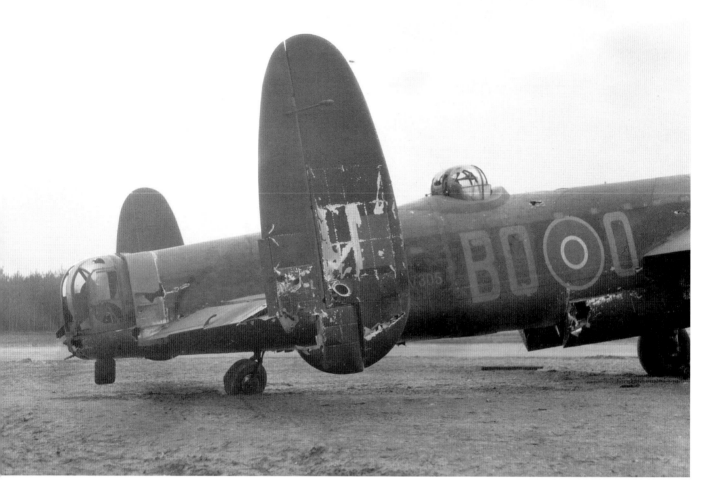

ABOVE What the British Army called shell shock in the First World War was often referred to by the Royal Air Force in the Second World War using the emotive term 'lacking moral fibre' – or LMF for short. Heavy bomber crews were susceptible to the effects of psychological stress owing to the intensity of operations and high casualty rates on the squadrons. This Avro Lancaster bomber was mauled by a German night-fighter over Berlin in an attack that left both gunners dead. *(Jonathan Falconer collection)*

Psychologists discovered, for instance, that gunners were more susceptible to combat stress than pilots because they viewed themselves as 'sitting ducks' in battle, while on the other hand the minds of pilots were focused on instrumentation and flying their aircraft. Research also validated the use of psychometric testing, with the Director of British Medical Services acknowledging:

In the end, it has been found that questions of air-sickness, injury and refusals, in effect preventable wastage, is largely bound up with the correct selection of officers and men [. . .] It has been said that one of the most striking features of British Airborne Divisions is the high esteem in which their medical services are held by the fighting troops and the active co-operation with them which is always present.[3]

Treatment of psychiatric problems within front-line medical units relied on basic and relatively simple 'PIES' principles. This acronym stood for: *proximity* – giving care near to the patient's combat unit; *immediacy* – treatment administered as soon as possible; *expectancy* – fostering the expectation of prompt return to combat duty; and *simplicity* – the notion that rest, recuperation, good hygiene and nourishment would go a long way to promoting recovery.

In theory, these principles still formed

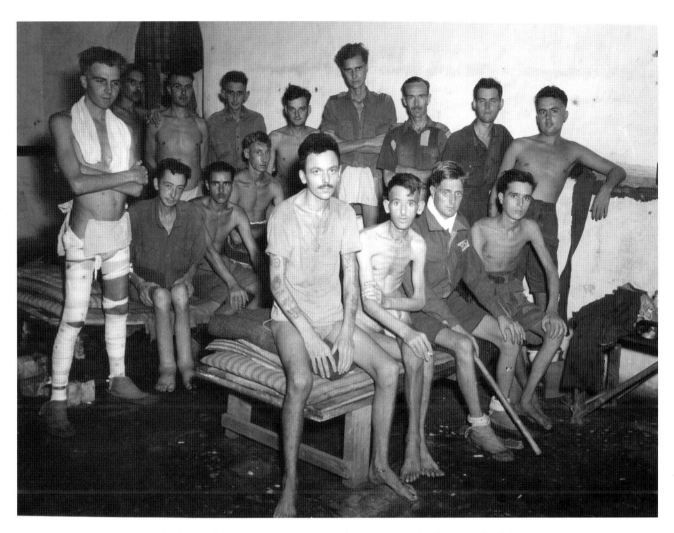

the bedrock of military psychiatric medicine during the Korean Conflict. A lack of front-line support in the early phase of the war, however, meant that in practice casualties displaying symptoms of anxiety, distress, panic, psychotic or dissociative states were usually evacuated from Pusan to Japan. This policy severely hampered recovery rates. For example, 1,800 psychiatric cases were sent to Japan over the course of three months in the summer of 1950. Only a handful of these returned to duty. Similarly, when battle-exhausted combatants in the 1st Marine Division were evacuated to hospital ships, very few returned to the front. Yet when members of this same division were treated near their unit with rest, sedation and psychological intervention, 50% were able to return to duty.[4]

British psychiatrists were also concerned that support was too far behind the lines to provide optimal care. They were particularly worried that

reservists, who were already disaffected, might succumb to disorders of the mind. Dr Flood, in charge of a 30-bed psychiatric unit in Kure, Japan, conducted a survey of British soldiers who were referred to him for assessment between December 1950 and November 1951. During this period 554 soldiers were referred and 365 were returned to duty.[5]

Most of those referred were suffering from mild cases of acute anxiety. Worries about family at home preoccupied some, while others complained of associated physical ailments such as headaches and indigestion. Some were suffering the after-effects of concussion. Soldiers experiencing more severe anxiety states displayed terror-stricken facial expressions and a heightened degree of panic-induced startle reflexes. These were treated with barbiturates and drug-induced narcosis. Depressive patients, meanwhile, refused to eat, were tearful and

ABOVE
**Psychologically
traumatised survivors
of a Japanese
POW Camp.**
*(Jonathan Falconer
collection)*

DIAGNOSTIC BREAKDOWN OF PSYCHIATRIC CASUALTIES IN UK ELEMENTS OF KOREAN FORCE BETWEEN DECEMBER 1950 AND NOVEMBER 1951

Anxiety states	287
Hysteria	73
Maladjusted and psychopathic personalities and dullards	42
Schizophrenia	22 & (?4)
Organic reactive psychosis	1
Manic-depressive psychosis	7
NAD (No abnormality detected)	118

Source: J.J. Flood, 'Psychiatric Casualties in UK Elements of Korean Force December 1950–November 1951', *Journal of Royal Army Medical Corps* 100-01-04 (1 January 1954).

in many instances non-communicative. The most impressive 'cure' rate could be found among the hysterics, many of whom responded positively to abreaction treatment. Interestingly, members of the Royal Navy and RAF were excluded from Flood's survey because the incidence of psychiatric disturbance in these sections of the armed forces was negligible.

Numbers of psychiatric casualties ebbed and flowed depending on the intensity of fighting. Military offensives accompanied by increased mortar fire led to an influx of battle-exhausted casualties, and to some extent associations between psychiatric disorders and issues of malingering persisted. Soldiers were accused of deliberately getting frostbite by removing footwear in the extreme cold of Korean winters, and physical conditions were often dismissed as psychosomatic. Flood was quick to point out, however, that such cases should be approached and treated with at least two sessions of psychotherapy.

It is quite certain that a soldier who can externalise his anxieties to an ear which he recognises as being both sympathetic and firm derives considerable benefit. His anxiety is predominantly the fear of personality disintegration in the face of danger rather than any specific fear of death, maiming or captivity by his enemy, and it was invariably on this theme that psychotherapy is gainfully rendered.[6]

Nevertheless, the Assistant Director of Medical Services, Colonel Morgan-Smith, cautioned military psychiatrists against dismissing physical manifestations of illness when they were presented within a psychological context, stating: 'Chronic low back pain, gastro-intestinal disturbances and vasomotor symptoms were often bodily responses to anxiety, resentment or low morale.'[7]

By this stage war neurosis was recognised as a genuine condition, but it remained a contentious issue. When compiling a standard reference textbook for psychiatrists in 1952, the American Psychiatric Association alluded to the possibility of 'gross stress reactions' in terms of temporary responses to environmental stress but failed to list war neurosis as a disorder. Believing 'gross stress' to be a fleeting aberration of normal psychological function, association members were convinced that victims made a full recovery as soon as they were removed from environmental stress.[8] Moreover, in some instances psychological disorders continued to be misdiagnosed as psychosomatic illnesses.

The subsequent experiences of combatants in Vietnam, however, left little doubt as to the existence of combat stress. Even the widespread use of newly developed, powerful anti-psychotic drugs such as phenothiazine and chlorpromazine could not hide the psychological trauma of those deployed in this drawn-out conflict. In many respects these medications represented a major turning point in psychiatric care, allowing patients who had been previously institutionalised to return to their homes and communities. US military psychiatrists nonetheless spoke out against what they saw as an over-reliance on these new pharmaceuticals in Vietnam, some strongly hinting at an unethical wartime military–industrial financial alliance.[9]

Psychological disturbances in US troops were compounded by easy access to recreational drugs and alcohol. Lysergic acid diethylamide (LSD) was popular, along with marijuana and heroin. Dysfunctional behaviour patterns caused by drug dependency therefore became intertwined with psychological reactions to the bloody reality of war.

Psychiatrist Robert Lifton, a veteran of the Korean War acknowledged: 'Warfare produces an advanced state of psychic numbing to images of death, destruction, and actions of general brutalisation.'[10]

Military psychiatrists, along with religious padres, did their utmost to support troops in the face of unpredictable, sinister guerrilla warfare. Sports and entertainment events were introduced to improve morale and group cohesion and good communication skills were emphasised in training sessions. Talking

BELOW Vietnam veterans continued to live with PTSD long after the war had finished. *(Copyright unknown)*

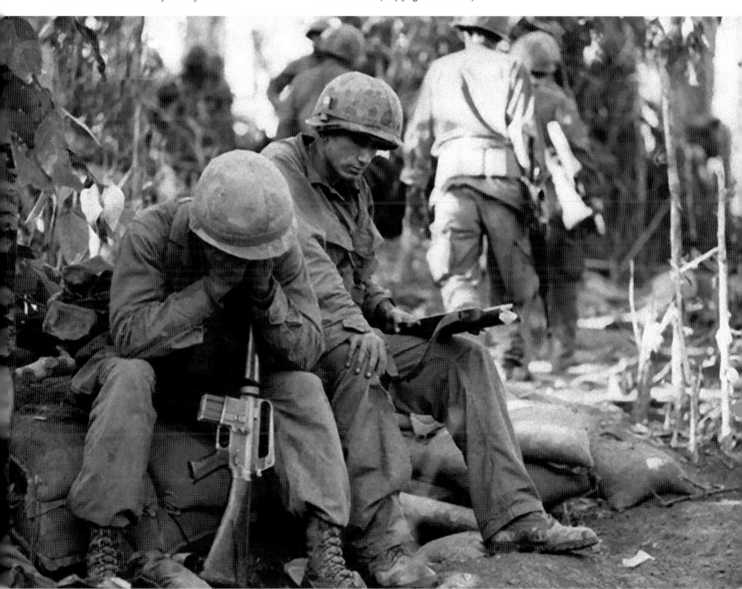

therapies – believed to release repressed emotions – were frequently implemented, and unit identification was emphasised. Despite these interventions, cases of battle exhaustion/war neurosis continued to rise at an alarming rate. Disciplinary cases relating to alcohol and drug abuse also increased. Psychiatrists began to describe the catatonic 'thousand-yard stare' of mentally detached soldiers, who no longer cared about their fellow human beings, their surroundings or their own well-being: soldiers devoid of all emotional life or connection with humankind.

Psychological problems could creep up on veterans unexpectedly in later life. As a retired surgeon who served in Vietnam acknowledged, psychological trauma was not an easy condition to live with:

When I told a Veterans Affairs psychologist that I did not think my late in life symptoms were related to my Vietnam experience, he smiled. "If you really believe that you were not affected by running into a minefield, disarming a disturbed soldier while he was

threatening to shoot you, and watching your patients die while you treated them in mud and under fire – you are an idiot."[11]

On their return home, Vietnam veterans frequently exhibited stress-related symptoms, including drug and alcohol abuse, an inability to stay in employment or maintain healthy relationships, irritability, antisocial behaviour, clinical depression, flashbacks, sleep deprivation, periods of psychosis, oversensitisation, anxiety disorders and anger management issues. Collectively these symptoms became known as post-Vietnam syndrome – a condition largely overlooked by existing veteran associations. Set against the tumultuous political background of civil rights movements and anti-war demonstrations, veterans received little compassion for their plight. Anti-war protestors even accused them of being traitors. Despite the compelling testimonies of military psychiatrists, it was not until 1979 that all veterans were given access to counselling services.

The following year the American Psychiatric Association, updating its textbook, *Diagnostics and Statistics Manual of Mental Disorders*, coined the term 'post-traumatic stress disorder' for the first time. No longer seen as a temporary aberration, war neurosis was officially recognised as a serious and life-debilitating mental disorder. No longer blighted by associations with malingering, this monumental shift in US psychiatric attitudes was a direct result and legacy of the psychological trauma inflicted on combatants during the Vietnam War.

There was also a growing recognition that the role of psychiatrists and chaplains/padres overlapped. Reporting from the Falklands Campaign it was noted that:

Interesting in its unexpectedness was the account of the role of a psychiatrist and no less interesting was the way in which he and his staff undertook with success much of the work traditionally associated with chaplains to the forces, about whom nothing was said. Men grieve for fallen comrades and lost ships and they need to be encouraged to say so; little may need to be said in return and tears should be regarded as evidence not of

BELOW A female military therapist counsels a military veteran. Attitudes towards PTSD have changed substantially and combatants experiencing symptoms are encouraged to come forward and obtain treatment. *(Getty Images)*

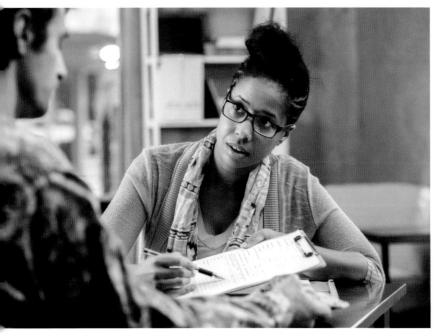

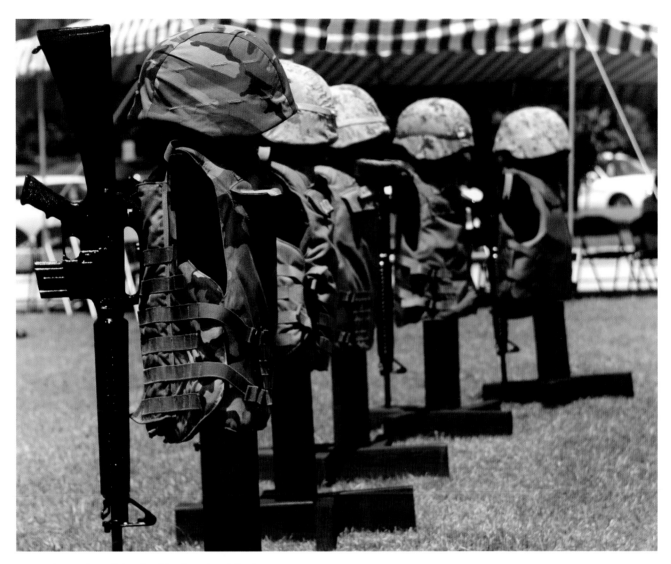

weakness but of depth of feeling. A soldier in tears may be an upsetting sight but it should move the observer to sympathy.[12]

For many Marines, however, humour was a saving grace – however dark. A patient named Chopsy Gray was hit by a blast and fragments of a mortar bomb that had landed beside him. 'The impact tore his right leg off and perforated the other limb with many metal fragments. Apparently, he had then shouted out: "I've lost me f****** leg!", to which a rather laconic reply from behind a nearby clump of tussock grass was: "No you haven't, Chopsy – it's landed over here . . .".'[13]

On another occasion, after a particularly gruelling field hospital shift, Rick Jolly poured out 'Arduous Duty' tots of whisky for the Army and rum for the Jack and Royal. One Marine looked up and said: 'Cheers Boss! Bloody good wet that – and now we've done the practical, any chance of getting the theory some time?'[14]

Giving combatants an opportunity to talk about their experiences was shown to mitigate the effects of combat stress. Rick Jolly observed in the aftermath of the Falklands:

If a group of marines wanted to stay up all night and talk about shared experiences, that was fine – as long as they all 'turned to' next morning. If someone wanted to curl up in his cabin all day, missing meals while mourning a dead friend, well that was fine too – as long as good order as an extension of self-discipline was maintained. There was a happy, vibrant atmosphere aboard the ship. Recreation expanded to fill the time available. In slow time, the Royal Marines of 3 Commando Brigade were decompressing steadily after their short but intense experiences of war. This gradual release of tension and pressure was all a happy accident, because it really was the best way of staving off development of a corrosive set of symptoms called post-traumatic stress disorder. The benefit of sharing memories and recalling emotions honestly, in the company of those who had been through the same experiences as you, brought with it an understanding that your reactions were completely normal.[15]

A fundamental acceptance of the causes of psychological trauma and how to mitigate against it, was beginning to surface. In the years following the First Iraq War the US Defense Department made concerted efforts to identify those members of the military who were most at risk of developing PTSD. The Millennium Cohort project studied 150,000 members in all sections of the US forces in the late 1990s. The study was the first of its kind to link detailed lifestyle choices, baseline health statistics and deployment information to a wide array of electronic databases. Initial research outcomes suggested that PTSD rates were directly linked to combat exposure rather than simply being deployed in a combat zone.[16]

Follow-up research into the lives and mental health of the US Millennium Cohort continue to look at the personal and strategic implications of PTSD, but attempts to devise a standard approach to deal with psychological trauma was pioneered by the British Royal Marines. Entitled Trauma Risk Management (TRiM), the system is a post-trauma event protocol aimed at reducing the effects of combat stressors. In addition to comprehensive self-help guidelines, TRiM also advises relatives of PTSD sufferers to do the following: listen carefully, spend time with the traumatised person, offer their assistance and a listening ear even if they have not asked for help, reassure them, help them with everyday tasks, allow them some private time

BELOW Post-traumatic stress disorder poster. *(US Air Force photo)*

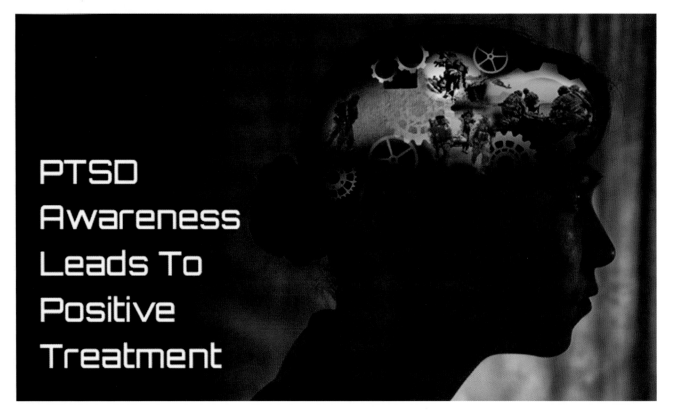

PTSD Awareness Leads To Positive Treatment

and not to take their anger or other feelings personally. More importantly, TRiM cautions relatives: do not tell them that 'they are lucky it was not worse', or 'you will get over it' or to 'pull yourself together'; these statements do not console traumatised people. Instead, tell them that you recognise an event has occurred and that you want to understand and assist them.[17]

Further military research has revealed the efficacy of regular debriefing sessions throughout deployment periods to prevent mental overload and improve unit identities. Known as battle-mind principles, debriefings stress the need for strong psychological focus, unwavering trust in military leaders and training, the importance of comradeship and the physiology of PTSD. Combatants are also introduced to role-playing scenarios and instructed in cognitive methods, which reduce anxiety levels and improve individual resilience. In recent years psychologists and psychiatrists alike have advocated the use of stress inoculation therapies prior to deployment to combat zones. The notion that the mind can be inoculated against trauma in the same way as the body can be inoculated against disease is radical, but effective. Stress inoculation therapy is particularly useful for combat medics who are regularly confronted with horrific and mentally disturbing injuries.

Within the US Army research facilities, high-fidelity simulators have been produced to prepare medics for combat zones. Imitating the sight, smell and feel of blast injuries they realistically re-create images encountered by battlefield medics.

The Multiple Amputation Trauma Trainer (MATT) developed under this initiative is a high-fidelity improvised explosive device (IED) blast injury simulator with state-of-the-art special effects, with sensing animatronics technologies to support haemorrhage control training, introduced movement for the first time, increasing realism and immersion to support stress inoculation training.[18]

For sufferers of PTSD, combinations of medication, counselling and post-traumatic support networks such as TRiM have improved outcomes significantly. But as American surgeon Paul Roach recalled, the sense of returning home after completing two tours of combat duty exacted a mental toll:

They say war is intoxicating, but it wasn't intoxicating for me. It's like the intensity and sharpness of the experience carved deep channels in my mind, and my thoughts as they flow about their daily business easily finding themselves rolling downstream into those channels. Since I've been back, I've been moulting, I suppose. I'm impacted but not injured. I've had up days and some down ones too. It's like there are these pockets of bubbles of overpowering emotion floating about in my life's arena, and when I'm not bopping into them and they're not bopping into me everything is fine, perfectly fine. But there you can be, marching along, doing your thing, and one of those little bubbles find you and 'pop' it bursts and for a little bit you're under its spell and you're right back in Afghanistan or more likely you are just getting emotional or tearing up for no reason. 'It's my allergies', I say as I excuse myself if there's someone around.[19]

The sheer weight of responsibility of a combat medic could also be found in: 'the soldier who kept seven or eight tourniquets on his arms, so every time he flexed his arms, he could feel them clumped there, could still feel them there after he came home, unscathed physically. Still prepared even in a time and place when he doesn't need to be, still in his head in the war.'[20]

Deployment and post-deployment data has revealed that some victims of PTSD, especially those wounded in explosions who sustained a TBI, have deteriorated dramatically with the progression of time. Furthermore, in many respects investigations into this phenomenon has come full circle. With the contemporary discovery of previously undetected cell abnormalities within the brains of blast victims, research has recently revisited earlier First World War notions of war neurosis. Scientists may yet prove a connection between the shell-shock sufferers of over a hundred years ago and current blast victims with PTSD.

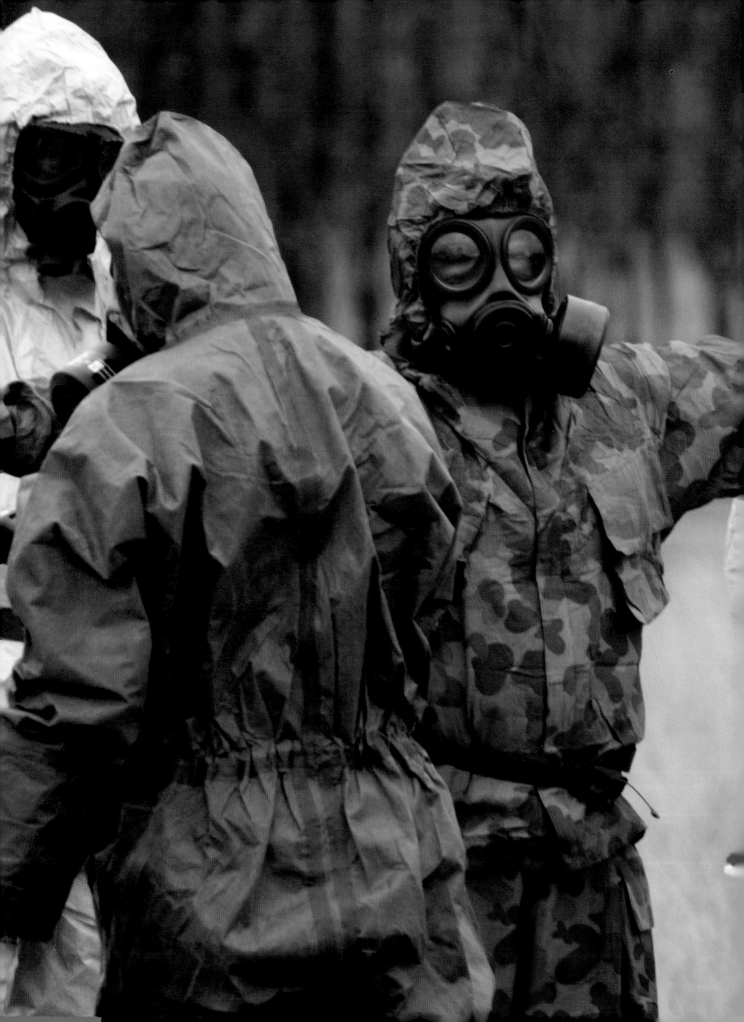

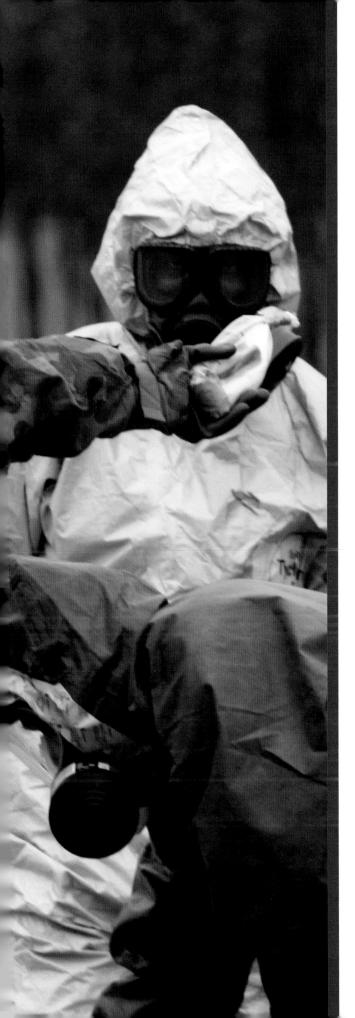

Chapter Nine

Chemical, biological, radiological and nuclear weapons (CBRN)

The prevention of CBRN attacks is dependent on military medical intelligence. Treatment and care of CBRN victims is guided by NATO mass casualty principles of medical management.

These include decontamination guidelines, strict evaluation of water and food supply chains, and the safe disposal of dead bodies.

OPPOSITE An Australian Army officer is checked for signs of contamination during a chemical weapons inspection in September 2010. *(Commonwealth of Australia)*

145

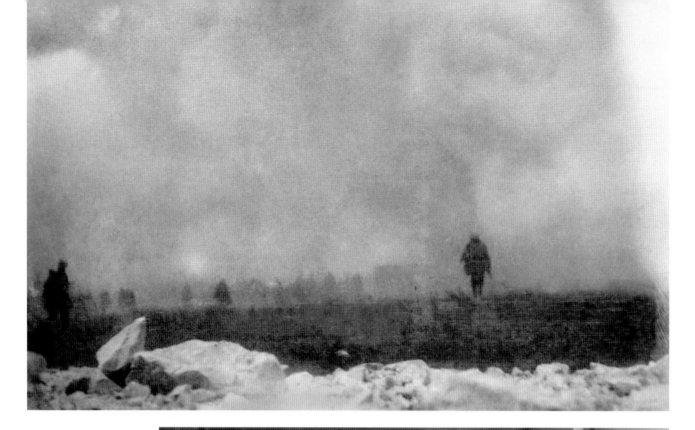

ABOVE British troops advance through a cloud of poison gas on the opening day of the Battle of Loos, 25 September 1915. This remarkable photograph was taken from the trench which they have just left by a soldier of the London Rifle Brigade.

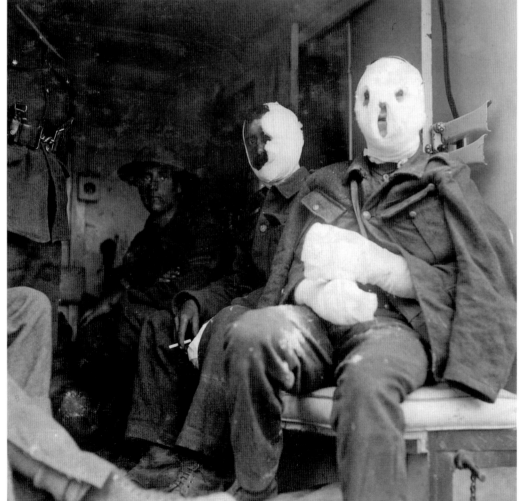

RIGHT Having received initial treatment at a casualty clearing station on the Western Front, soldiers injured by mustard gas wait to be transferred to a general hospital for further treatment.

(Copyright unknown)

Chemical, biological, radiological and nuclear weapons (CBRN) can rapidly kill thousands, inflict massive casualties, destroy buildings, terrain and equipment and severely disrupt tactical military missions. Known as weapons of mass destruction from the outset, they have become the most feared of all, even though they arguably represent the most spineless methods of waging war. As British General Sir Charles Ferguson pointed out during the First World War, chemical warfare is the most cowardly of all forms of warfare, since the ordinary fighting man, however brave, has no chance when faced with insidious gas attacks or similar sinister threats.

Following the first gas attacks in 1915, Dr Harvey Cushing described the anguish of victims on the Western Front:

When we got back to the ambulance, the air was full of tales of asphyxiating gas which the Germans had turned loose – but it is difficult to get a straight story. A huge, low-lying greenish cloud of smoke with a yellowish top began to roll down from German trenches, fanned by a steady easterly wind. At the same time there was a terrifically heavy bombardment. The smoke was suffocating and smelled to some like ether and sulphur, to another like a thousand sulphur matches, to still another like burning rosin. Only sixty men out of a thousand survived the attack. Later I saw a number of recently gassed cases – two of them still conscious, but gasping, livid and about to die, and I hope they didn't have long to wait poor chaps. Then we saw many of the severely gassed men who had come in this morning – terrible business – one man as blue as a sailor's serge, simply pouring out with every cough a thick albuminous secretion, and too busy fighting for air to bother much about anything else – a most horrible form of death for a strong man.[1]

In response to gas attacks a British physician named J.S. Haldane, working with C.G. Douglas, L. Hill and J. Barcroft, developed an effective gas mask, or respirator. Haldane, who had first identified the fact that Germans were using chlorine and phosgene in their arsenal of gas canisters, conducted several experiments. He would sit in a sealed room while various gases were poured in through a door. Haldane would note how these gases affected his brain function and respiration. Chlorine and phosgene worked by causing mass inflammation and irritation of the lungs, which in turn caused oxygen deprivation. Haldane concluded that lungs affected in this way needed to be flooded with oxygen as soon as possible after a gas attack. Subsequently he constructed special apparatus designed to administer oxygen to soldiers affected in this way. Clinical trials were performed on gas victims with encouraging results, and eventually over 4,000 oxygen cylinders were sent to base hospitals in France. Thus, oxygen therapy became a new and accepted method of treatment for gas victims and more men survived attacks.

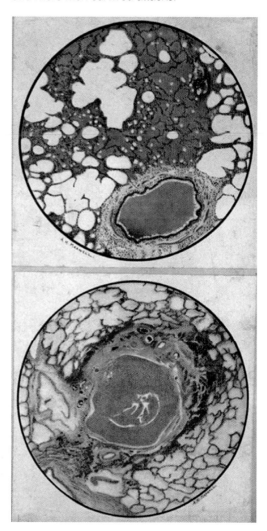

LEFT Microscopic section of human lung tissue from mustard gas poisoning, with death at the end of the second day. *(Wellcome Collection CC-BY)*

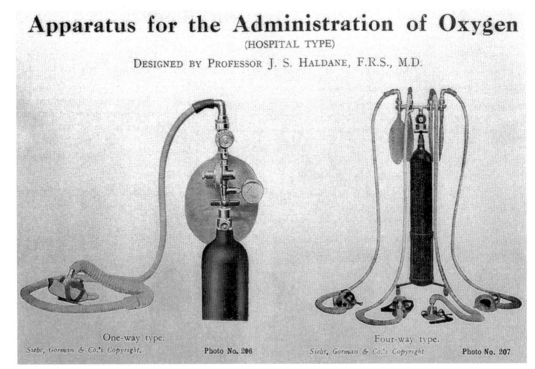

DEFINITIONS OF CBRN WEAPONS

Chemical hazards – any toxic chemical manufactured, used, transported or stored which can cause death or harm through exposure. This includes chemical weapon agents and chemicals developed or manufactured for use in industrial operations or research that pose a hazard, are collectively characterised as Toxic Industrial Chemicals (TIC).

Biological hazards include any organism, or substance derived from an organism, that poses a threat to the health of any living organism. Biological hazards are a threat to conducting military operations. This can include medical waste, samples of a micro-organism, virus or toxin (from a biological source) that can impact on human health and spread infectious disease. Biological material that is manufactured, used, transported or stored by industrial, medical or commercial processes, which could pose an infectious or toxic threat, are collectively characterised as Toxic Industrial Biologicals (TIB).

Radiological hazards include ionising radiation that can cause damage, injury or destruction from either external irradiation or radiation from radioactive materials within the body. Radiological material that is manufactured, used, transported or stored by industrial, medical or commercial processes are collectively characterised as Toxic Industrial Radiological (TIR).

Nuclear hazards are those dangers associated with the over-pressure, thermal and radiation effects from a nuclear explosion. Nuclear hazards come from the employment of nuclear weapons and devices that can generate radiation; low altitude; nuclear air burst shock waves; severe winds; electro-magnetic pulse (EMP); and intense heat that can cause casualties and damage through burning, crushing, bending, tumbling, breaking, penetrating debris and residual radiation in the form of fall-out.

Source: *Operations in Chemical, Biological, Radiological and Nuclear Environments.* Joint publication 3-11, US Joint Chiefs of Staff, 29 October 2018.

During the Second World War, Germans systematically used poison gases to kill millions of Jews and developed the highly toxic nerve agent tabun. Japan's biological warfare against China inflicted plague, cholera and typhus on an unsuspecting Chinese population, in addition to numerous instances of medical experimentation. As British Prime Minister Churchill asserted:

a study of disease – of pestilence methodically prepared and deliberately launched upon man and beast is certainly being pursued in the laboratories of more than one great country. Blight to destroy crops, anthrax to slay horses and cattle, plague to poison not armies but whole districts – such are the lines along which military science is remorselessly advancing.

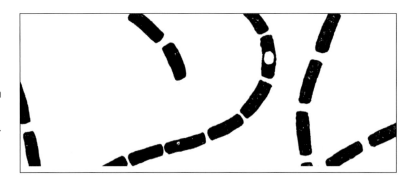

ABOVE Bacilli of anthrax. Perhaps the most feared of all biological weapons, anthrax can infect people via the skin, respiratory tract and by injection. If spores are released into the air people are likely to contract anthrax by inhalation and over 80% will die as a result. Used by the German Army in the First World War to infect cattle and animal feed destined for consumption by Allied personnel, anthrax has a long history as a biological weapon. *(Wellcome Collection CC-BY)*

Subsequently, the US decision to drop atom bombs on Hiroshima and Nagasaki in 1945 signalled the arrival of a new and terrifying age of destructive weaponry. Capable of wiping out humanity with unprecedented ease, nuclear bombs created a shadow of uncertainty across the globe, and the post-war nuclear arms race became symbolic of the Cold War era. Furthermore, in the early days of testing hydrogen bombs, scientists appeared oblivious of the long-term effects caused by radiation and fallout. Therefore, soldiers who were ordered to watch nuclear tests in the 1950s were told to simply cover their eyes and hit the ground face down as bombs were detonated. Years later these same soldiers suffered with a variety of cancers, predominantly lymphoma. Civilians living downwind of testing sites suffered from similar conditions, and there was little anyone could do to remedy this situation. Even the Atom Bomb Casualty Commission was more concerned with observing the after-effects of nuclear testing on survivors than it was in providing any effective treatment.

In the following years, in terms of prevention, detection, triage and treatment, CBRN posed unique challenges for combat medics. In Korea many US deployed soldiers had already witnessed nuclear testing but did not necessarily exhibit the health problems associated with fallout, whereas chemical warfare waged in Vietnam had both instant and latent detrimental effects on military and civilian health. As US jets dumped huge quantities of napalm across the country, doctors were initially at a loss as to how to treat its victims. Napalm was made from petrochemicals which stuck to skin and burned soft tissue down to the bone. Nurses removed the dead skin of napalm victims while they were immersed in saline 'burn baths'. Once this process was complete, doctors set to work painstakingly creating skin grafts. However, in patients with over 30% burns, skin grafts were often unsuccessful.

The use of mass pesticide and herbicides between 1961 and 1971 created further problems. During this period more than 20.2 million gallons of military herbicides were used to defoliate forests and mangroves in what was then South Vietnam to deny cover to enemy troops and make bombing targets more visible.[2] Once considered to be safe, the most notable of these herbicides was known as Agent Orange. Like other herbicides used at this time, Agent Orange contained dioxin, a highly toxic substance which caused significant health problems for military personnel in Vietnam and the indigenous population. Dioxin interferes with the metabolism of porphyrins (and the main symptom of poisoning is derived from an increase of porphyrins in the organism – *ie*, porphyria cutanea tarda) by induction of delta aminolevulate synthetase. Dioxin also has carcinogenic, hepatotoxic, nephrotoxic, teratogenic and

DISEASES FOR WHICH MILITARY SERVICE IN VIETNAM MAY BE CONSIDERED PRESUMPTIVE OF EXPOSURE BY THE DEPARTMENT OF VETERANS AFFAIRS FOR THE PURPOSE OF TREATMENT AND COMPENSATION

- Amyloid light-chain amyloidosis
- Chronic B-cell leukaemias
- Chloracne
- Diabetus [*sic*] mellitus type 2
- Hodgkin's disease
- Ischaemic heart disease
- Multiple myeloma
- Non-Hodgkin's lymphoma
- Parkinson's disease
- Peripheral neuropathy, early onset

- Porphyria cutanea tarda
- Prostate cancer
- Respiratory cancers, including lung
- Soft tissue sarcomas (other than osteosarcoma, chondrosarcoma, Kasoi's sarcoma and mesothelioma)
- Spina bifida in offspring.

Source: US Department of Veterans Affairs, https://www. publichealth.va.gov/exposures/agentorange/conditions/asp.

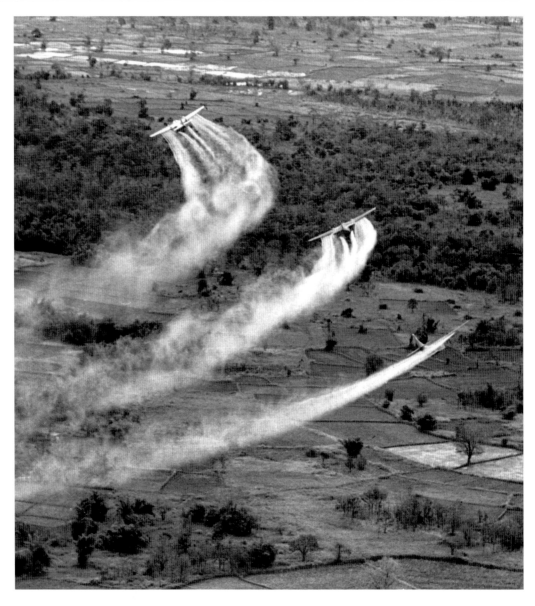

RIGHT Vietnam War defoliation mission – Fairchild UC-123 Provider military transport aircraft spray Agent Orange over the South Vietnamese countryside. As part of Operation Ranch Hand, US Air Force helicopters and aircraft were fitted with chemical tanks and spray bars to release defoliants and herbicides over rural areas to deprive the Viet Cong of food and vegetation cover. *(Shutterstock)*

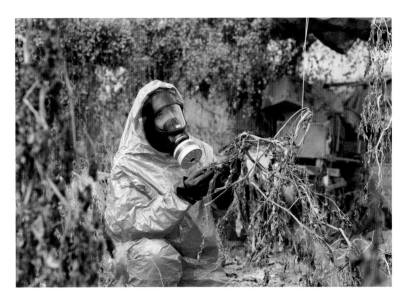

RIGHT Day after – portrait of a man wearing German protection clothes against radiation, biological and chemical substances. He is analysing dead plants for evidence of biological or chemical warfare or nuclear accident.

(Getty Images)

embryotoxic effects and causes dermal changes. There is no specific antidote, making treatment very difficult and symptomatic. The effects of dioxin following acute administration are relatively delayed, which is a limiting factor in its use as a chemical weapon.[3]

Not wholly content with the effects of chemical warfare in terms of flushing out the enemy, there were some US commanders who mooted the idea of a nuclear alternative to the Vietnam stalemate, though a Central Intelligence Agency memorandum dated 18 March 1966 highlighted the drawbacks of taking such a radical course of action. Two years later, despite concerted efforts by General Westmoreland to gain approval for nuclear weapons in Vietnam, President Johnson, fearing Chinese intervention, dismissed such a strategy.[4] From a military medical standpoint, dealing with massive casualties in the wake of a nuclear conflict was unimaginable. Since residual radiation could not be eliminated, other strategies employed to protect personnel simply relied on restricting the time they were exposed to radiation, increasing their distance away from radioactive sources and putting up physical barriers if available.

With an increasing reliance on chemical weapons in Vietnam, military scientists explored the possibility of antidotes and post-exposure treatments. Chemical agents usually worked by inducing disruption of the nervous system, causing systemic blistering, uncontrollable choking or vomiting, precipitated breathing difficulties, bleeding or crying (CS/tear gas). All were able to incapacitate victims within a short space of time. But since tear gas and similar chemicals were used primarily for civilian crowd control, military personnel focused on protecting troops against the disabling, life-threatening capabilities of blister and nerve agents. VX,

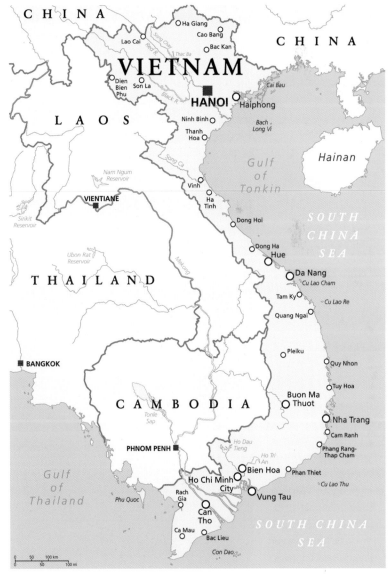

RIGHT North and South Vietnam. *(Shutterstock)*

Sarin (GB), Soman (GD) and Tabun (GA), were the most routinely used nerve agents and acted by severely interrupting nerve function, causing seizures, paralysis and death. Indeed, British serviceman Ronald Maddison died in 1953 after being deliberately exposed to Sarin during a scientific experiment conducted at the UK Defence Science and Technology centre at Porton Down. Nerve agents were used in liquid or gas forms and exhibited diverse levels of persistency. VX for instance was a persistent agent, while Sarin remained non-persistent.

Persistent agents were able to penetrate many substances, and victims could only be cared for by personnel wearing full barrier and respiratory protection. Absorbed through the lungs, mucous membranes and the skin, the effects of VX and Sarin were dose-dependent. With a lethal dose prompting symptoms in less than 60 seconds, death was likely to occur within five minutes. This gave medics little time to administer the antidote atropine. No medical vaccination programmes existed to protect against chemical weapons, but from 1990 onwards, administering pyridostigmine before deployment offered some pre-exposure protection against nerve agents.

Mustard, meanwhile, was the most popular choice of blister agents, absorbed through the skin, mucous membranes and lungs. Inflicting serious chemical burns on exposed skin or tissue, symptoms of mustard poisoning normally surfaced several hours after exposure. Capable of damaging any bodily tissue structure, inhalation of a blister agent could lead to fatal pneumonia. Blindness could occur in circumstances where eyes were exposed to mustard, and skin grafts were necessary in severe cases. Blister agents were traditionally disseminated as liquids or gases and lingered for weeks or months in the exposure area. Even during the First World War mustard gas stayed on the ground for a long time after its release, and anyone touching the skin or clothing of an affected person also became contaminated. Some victims initially displayed very little in the way of symptoms but later died of blistered lungs and enlarged hearts. Indeed, it was not unusual for men to die two or three weeks after contamination. Victims usually suffered from swelling of their throats and lungs, and a distinctive widespread rash of tiny purple bruises. Larger patches of bruising were also visible in areas where clothing

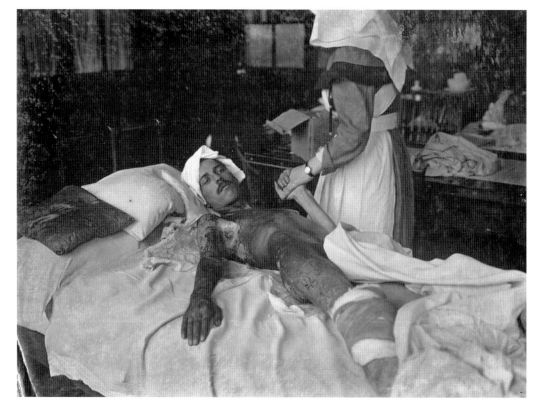

RIGHT Sawyer Spence, who suffered extensive mustard gas blisters on the Western Front in August 1918, undergoes treatment at Trent Bridge Hospital, Nottingham.
(Jon Spence)

may have been tighter, such as soldiers' waistbands.[5] If victims were able to access medical facilities quickly, then flooding the lungs with oxygen achieved positive results. But almost 100% of such gas victims continued to suffer impaired lung function and chronic bronchitis long after the war had ended. In subsequent conflicts mustard agents were deployed as liquids, because unpredictable changes in wind direction often blew gas back towards those who had released the weapon. The ability of a mustard agent to penetrate many layers of materials posed considerable problems. Special filtration technology and barrier suits were the only protection against this persistent substance.[6]

Blood agents, however, differed from nerve and blister chemical weapons by preventing the body's ability to use oxygen. Usually absorbed through the lungs or mucous membranes, victims of these agents displayed symptoms very quickly post-exposure. If available, medication was dispensed for treatment, but casualties were normally able to eliminate these toxic substances independently. In cases of severe exposure, assisted ventilation was occasionally required.

Biological weapons, meanwhile, presented combat medics with other problems. Unlike the flash of a nuclear explosion, or the sudden onset of violent symptoms indicative of chemical warfare, biological agents took a few days to incubate. Moreover, symptoms could very easily mimic naturally occurring epidemics. Therefore, even when numerous casualties appeared to be suffering with the same symptoms at the same time this did not necessarily point to a biological attack. Medics were instructed to look for evidence of diseases not associated with the geographical region, strains of antibiotic resistant viruses/bacteria and unusual clinical appearance. In circumstances where a biological attack was strongly suspected laboratory diagnosis was crucial. Everyone arriving at a field hospital from the contaminated area was treated as though contaminated. They were then stripped of their contaminated clothing and showered with large quantities of water or hypochlorite solution (0.5%). Depending on the presence of other injuries, emergency medical

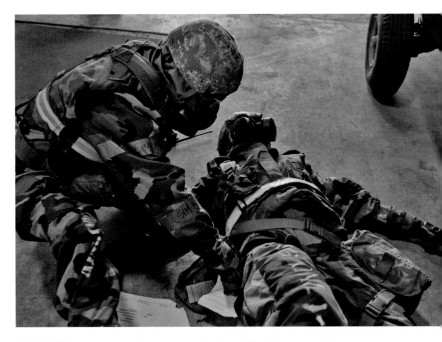

ABOVE US airmen practise giving antidotes. *(US Air Force photo)*

BELOW To protect RAF aircrew against chemical and biological agents, the Aircrew Respirator Mk 5 was introduced in 1969. It comprised a single-piece rubber hood and a heavy but flexible rubber cowl with neck seal worn over a single-piece under suit made from impregnated charcoal. Blown, filtered air was fed into the cowl to maintain a positive pressure, which prevented the entry of chemical or biological agents. *(Jonathan Falconer collection)*

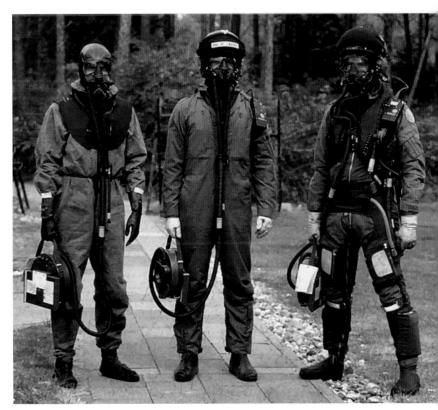

treatment was sometimes necessary before the decontamination process could begin, or in some cases carried out simultaneously. Maintaining respiration and stemming blood flow was a priority and for many casualties ventilation was assisted by mechanical means. Chemical agents were occasionally used in conjunction with biological and conventional weapons; in this scenario decontamination of chemical agents took precedence over those suffering from biological attacks.

Common biological weapons were divided between those with rapid-onset symptoms, such as the nerve agents, cyanide, mustard, lewisite and phosgene, and those with delayed-onset symptoms, like anthrax, smallpox, pneumonic plague, botulism and Q fever. Methods of transmission such as inhalation aerosol or cutaneous absorption also played a part in these time-frames. Various anti-toxins were available for specific conditions and intravenous antibiotics were administered as soon as possible, since most bacterial, chlamydial and rickettsial diseases responded to antibiotic therapy. Prophylactic antiviral drugs such as cidofovir were successfully used post-exposure against some viruses, for example smallpox, and ribavirin acted as a broad-spectrum antiviral therapy.[7]

Medics dealing with CBRN casualties needed to protect themselves as a priority,

both during and after the decontamination process, and initiate barrier nursing procedures to prevent cross-infection and further transmission of the biological agent. This policy protected non-contaminated personnel from those who were contaminated. Medics wore impermeable surgical gowns, gloves, oronasal masks, face shields or goggles and there were strict rules governing the observance of bodily fluids. Materials soiled by patient secretions and excreta, and samples for laboratory examination were all labelled as hazardous.[8] Spore-forming bacteria, for instance, could only be decontaminated by gamma-ray irradiation. Methods of disposing of contaminated remains were governed by NATO directives. Contaminated corpses were only the responsibility of medical personnel if patients died within the confines of medical systems; those fatally affected by biological warfare on the battlefield remained there, temporarily interred until further decontamination of the area was performed.

Victims of biological attacks came under NATO mass casualty principles of medical management, but unlike traditional wounds which required urgent and often extensive surgical procedures, biological agents usually produced severe respiratory paralysis, increasing demands for ventilators and other intensive-care machinery. Analgesia, reduction of body temperature in cases of fever, intravenous fluids with antibiotics/antivirals, the monitoring of blood gases and vital signs, along with barrier nursing techniques formed the basis of medical treatment. However, in circumstances where biological toxins were unleashed in large quantities, wider emergency control measures were implemented. Water supplies and food chains were safeguarded, the rodent and insect population restricted and civilian freedom of movement curtailed. Policies were implemented to prevent widespread panic and isolation shelters erected. The chances of surviving biological attacks varied according to preventive measures taken before deployment, and the agent used. Q fever, for example, was associated with low mortality rates, whereas yellow fever caused large numbers of fatalities.

To counteract this potential lottery of biological agents, combatants were usually

BELOW A US Air Force Senior Airman of the 60th Diagnostics and Therapeutics Squadron prepares a tray of specialised medical equipment ahead of an Yttrium-90 radio-embolisation procedure at Travis Air Force Base, California.
(US Air Force photo)

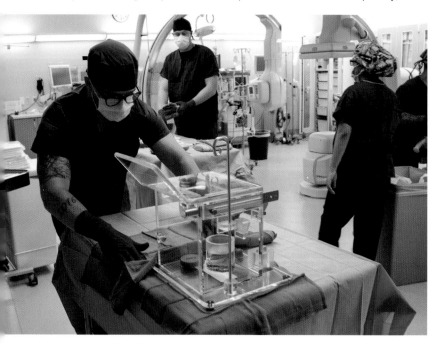

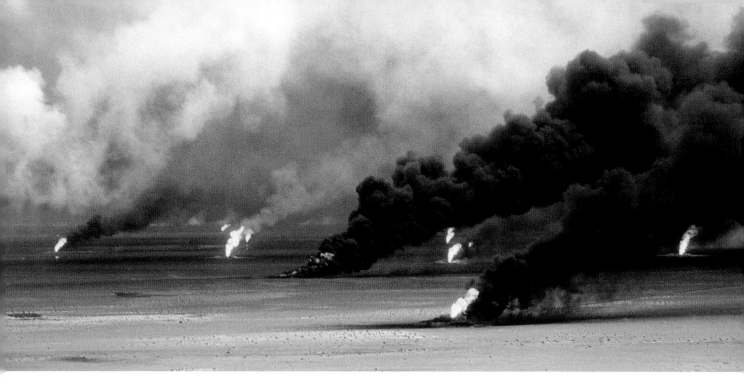

given a cocktail of immunisations prior to deployment. Before the Gulf War, US troops were immunised against anthrax, botulinum toxoid, smallpox, yellow fever, typhoid, cholera, hepatitis B, meningitis, whooping cough, polio and tetanus. Damaging military environmental exposures were listed as: burn pit smoke, water contaminated with benzene, trichloroethylene, vinyl chloride, endemic diseases, heat stroke/exhaustion, hexavalent chromium, mustard gas, nerve agents, pesticides, radiation (ionising and non-ionising), sand, dust, smoke and particulates.[9] In addition, chemoprophylaxis

and personal protective equipment was issued in preparation for CBRN warfare. Troops were instructed to wear battle dress over uniform, use high-efficiency particulate air masks (HEPA), protective gloves and over-boots. In 1993, however, the US general accounting office investigated chemical and biological detection capabilities and found that, at the outset of Operation Desert Storm, US military forces had the capability to detect all known Iraqi chemical agents and to warn its forces of an attack. Conversely, they had an extremely limited capability to detect biological threats.[10]

ABOVE Oil well fires rage outside Kuwait City in the aftermath of the First Gulf War. Retreating Iraqi troops set fire to Kuwait's oil fields, 21 March 1991. *(Shutterstock)*

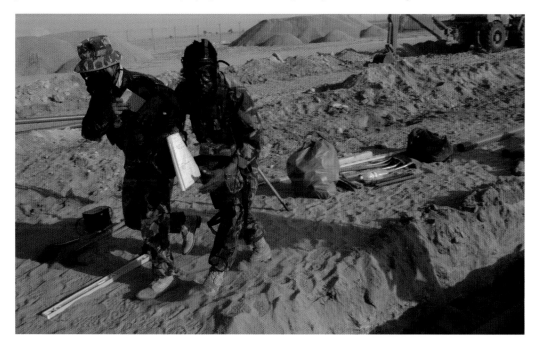

LEFT Members of 69 Gurkha Field Squadron, 36 Regiment, The Queen's Gurkha Engineers, assisting in the construction of a tented hospital abandon their work to run for cover after scrambling to put on gas masks during a Nuclear, Biological and Chemical Weapons alert. *(IWM OP-TELIC 03-010-08-167)*

155

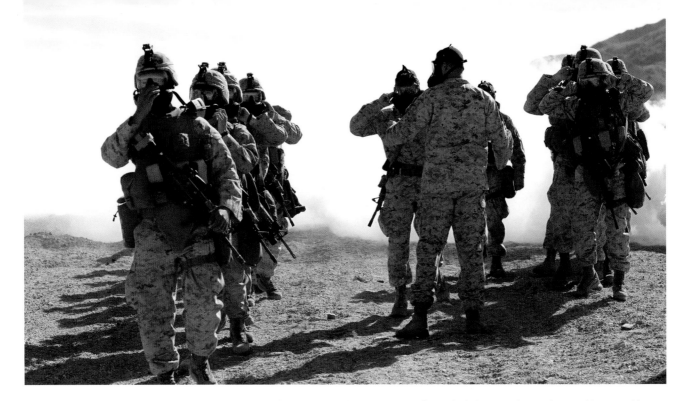

ABOVE US Marines and seamen take turns to march through a cloud of poison gas to test and become acquainted with their new CBRN gear at the Air Ground Combat Centre, Twenty-Nine Palms, California.
(Getty Images)

Immediately prior to Operation Iraqi Freedom, troops were prepared for all weapons of mass destruction from the outset. US and coalition forces wearing lightweight CBRN protective clothing performed numerous tactical exercises pre-deployment to ascertain levels of operational efficacy. Each suit contained an individual respirator protection system, and exposure to substances was recorded and monitored. The usual medical pre-deployment measures such as vaccinations and chemoprophylaxis, were supplemented by skin barrier sprays and repellents. Nerve agent pre-treatment sets (NAPS) and ComboPens containing atropine, P2S and avizafone were available as countermeasures to nerve agents, and doxycycline and ciprofloxacin were given in response to heightened threats of biological weapons. Collective Protection shelter systems (COLPRO) included air filtration mechanisms and air locks were used in the field to provide military personnel with hazard-free zones. From a medical management perspective, detailed preparation for a CBRN incident was crucial in terms of minimising risks of cross-contamination and for standardising logistical and treatment protocols.

However, CBRN victims presented unique problems in terms of care. Since they were often nursed within field hospitals already awash with wounded soldiers, staff and patients alike were either isolated or placed in quarantine.

Overwhelming numbers of casualties requiring intensive care facilities also placed a severe strain on hospitals. Moreover, decontamination procedures could prove difficult in cases where CBRN casualties had sustained wounds from conventional weapons. Hypochlorite solutions, used for decontamination for instance, could damage open wounds. Furthermore, evacuating victims, either from contaminated areas to places of safety, or from field hospitals to other medical facilities was difficult. Ideally the movement of contaminated patients and those infected with contagious biological agents was severely restricted in the first instance. Indeed, unless movement was essential to preserve life, limb or eyesight, or to maintain operational capabilities, evacuation was avoided. In cases where evacuation was considered medically necessary all efforts were focused on preventing the spread of contamination. Therefore, when evaluating the situation, combat medics were instructed to consider evacuation vehicles carefully, because some were much easier to decontaminate than others. Aeromedical evacuation from a CBRN environment, depending on the number and severity of casualties, had the potential to completely overwhelm aircraft capacity. In addition to massive numbers of casualties, the ensuing demand for specialised medical equipment, such as ventilators and intensive care equipment, potentially curtailed the size of military medical airlifts. The prospect of having to isolate patients with highly contagious biological contaminants also presented difficulties, although specialist aeromedical evacuation capabilities, such as those supplied by RAF CCAST, provide intensive care expertise for aeromedical evacuation of critically ill patients, including those on a ventilator. With the addition of an Air Transportable Isolator (ATI) RAF aeromedical teams can safely and efficiently transport a highly infectious patient if required.[11]

Ideally, however, senior military officials significantly reduce the risk of CBRN attacks by employing integrated preventive surveillance programmes to predict the use of weapons of mass destruction and implement protective countermeasures. Much of this surveillance work depends on the aspect of combat medicine known as military medical intelligence. As an essential component of strategic logistics, medical intelligence has played a pivotal role in the military planning of all conflicts. It is defined as that category of intelligence that stems from the collection, evaluation, analysis and interpretation of foreign medical, bio-scientific and environmental information that is of interest to strategic planning, and to military medical planning and operations for the conservation of the fighting strength of friendly forces and of the formation of assessments of foreign medical capabilities in both military and civilian sectors.[12] According to the US Joint Chiefs of Staff:

Accurate and timely medical intelligence is a critical medical tool, used to plan, execute and sustain military operations. A supporting intelligence element should exist at some point in the medical unit's chain of command. This element, whether military or civilian should be the primary source for the health services planner, to access the necessary intelligence for the execution of health services operations.[13]

Involving comprehensive health surveillance and meticulous recording of CBRN data, scientists work on early warning detection systems to alert combatants of incoming threats. Additionally, they discern atypical disease patterns, observe and document enemy

stockpiling of medical supplies and evaluate enemy medical treatment facilities.

The amassing of biological and chemical antidotes, for example, gives some indication of enemy intent to use CBRN. This surveillance combined with careful diagnostic testing in laboratories in the theatre of operations, enables the implementation of rapid countermeasures.

Identification of unusual strains of biological disease and current chemical weapons contribute to the development of new antidotes and vaccines, some of which can be auto-injected. In recent years there has been a proliferation of biological weapons, primarily because they are cheaper and easier to produce than their nuclear counterparts. This trend is of growing concern to those working within military and civilian healthcare systems, particularly in this current age of genetic engineering. In response to this increasing threat, scientists at Porton Down Defence Science and Technology Centre are constantly working to provide effective countermeasures to chemical and biological attacks.

BELOW Airmen from the 628th Medical Group and 375th Aeromedical Evacuation Squadron from Joint Air Base Charleston, South Carolina, and Scott Air Base III, transport a simulated patient during a training exercise during July 2018 at Joint Air Base Charleston. The goal of the training was to implement and evaluate the procedure of transportation for highly infectious patients from one location to another via aeromedical transportation. *(US Air Force photo)*

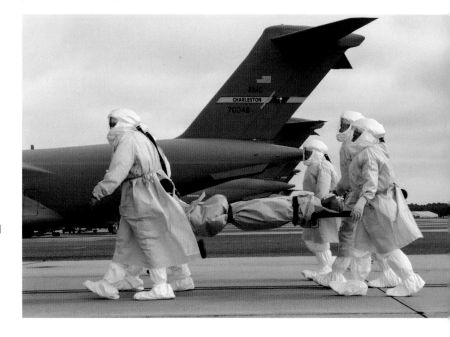

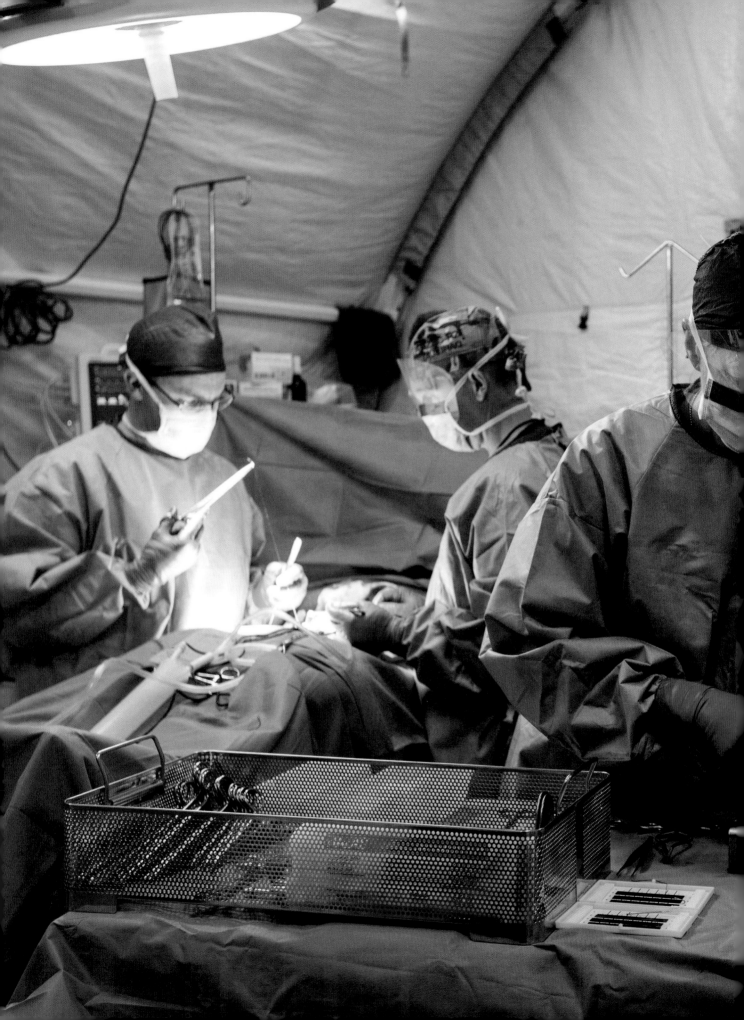

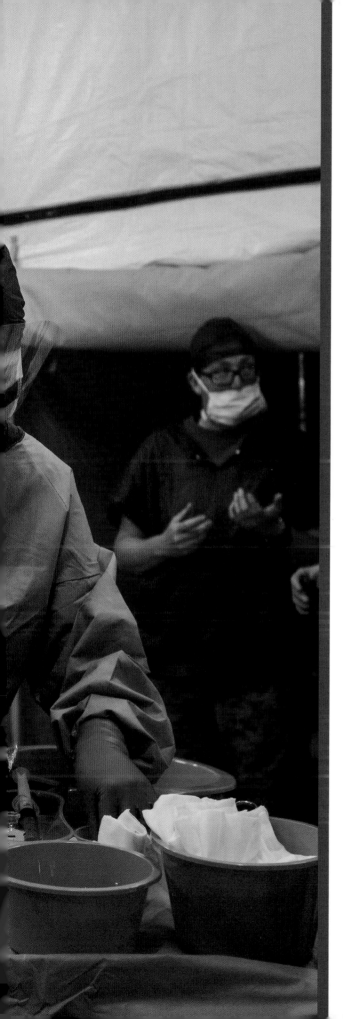

Chapter Ten

Focus on the field hospital

Mobile Army Surgical Hospitals (MASH) were introduced during the Korean War with great success. Yet field hospitals, static or mobile, came in many shapes and forms including tented accommodation, prefabricated buildings and disused refrigeration plants. All of these were staffed by highly skilled and devoted combat medics.

OPPOSITE A medical team comprising personnel from the Australian Army, Navy and Air Force perform an emergency procedure on an American soldier at the Taji military complex in Iraq. *(Commonwealth of Australia – Department of Defence)*

The history of the field hospital is as old as war itself. Fighting forces such as those organised by the Ancient Greeks and Romans all established some form of medical care for their warriors. Moreover, long before the emergence of germ theory in the late 19th century, military commanders had known not to camp near swamps or marshlands because of the risk of catching diseases such as typhoid or cholera from contaminated water. Theories such as miasma were rife and field hospital sites were chosen with care. They needed to be situated near clean water supplies and suitable transport networks for ease of casualty transfer.

Communication infrastructures were also important. Thus, British and French First World War field hospitals were based near railway sidings and reasonable roads, all of which linked up to major sea ports. The static nature of this conflict, however, enabled field hospitals to remain in place (unless flattened by bombs), for the duration of the war. Consisting of between 12 and 16 30-bed wards, at least 2 operating theatres, a laboratory and a pharmacy, these establishments were linked to forward field ambulances and casualty clearing stations. At this stage field hospitals also became hotbeds of medical research. Astute enough to realise that newly emerging medical problems could only be overcome by research and experimentation, Colonel Sir James Clark of the Order of St John field hospital established a medical research society in Étaples on 18 August 1915. He argued that 'members would need to initiate medical innovation and experimentation. They would have a God-given opportunity to not only be of service to their patients but also to make a phenomenal contribution to physiology, surgery and neurology.' The Director of Gas Services, C.H. Foulkes, shared Clark's view, pointing out: 'We have in the theatre of war itself a vast experimental ground [. . .] Human beings provide the material for these experiments on both sides of no-man's land.'[1]

Despite being overwhelmed with casualties on many an occasion, medical staff working in tented and prefabricated hospitals on the Western Front produced a plethora of research papers on a wide range of medical and surgical conditions. From investigations into disordered action of the heart to experimental brain surgery, surgeons and physicians alike collected statistics and published their research findings in leading medical journals. Indeed, the foundations of nearly all medical specialism were laid at this time, as staff simultaneously fought valiantly to save men from the ravages of war.

These static medical facilities quickly became small village-type communities, complete with a variety of social activities designed to maintain the morale of staff and patients. Theatrical groups, art and educational classes, choirs, chess clubs, ornithology lectures, gym, cricket and football teams were just some of the measures engineered to keep everyone from slowly sinking into an abyss dominated by blood, pus and bandages. When they were not dealing with a tidal wave of severely mutilated bodies, in off-duty hours staff would go for long walks or bicycle rides and gather for picnics on the beach or in the countryside. Outside the hospital attractive gardens were constructed where recovering soldiers could sit peacefully or stroll gently along narrow walkways. Unfortunately, these same gardens alerted enemy planes to the existence of Allied hospitals, and they became a target for aerial bombardment as a result.

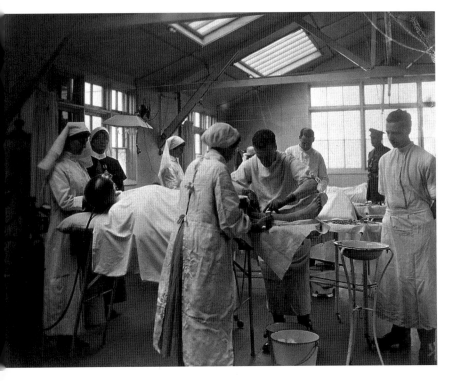

BELOW First World War British Army operating theatre near Boulogne. *(Wellcome Collection *

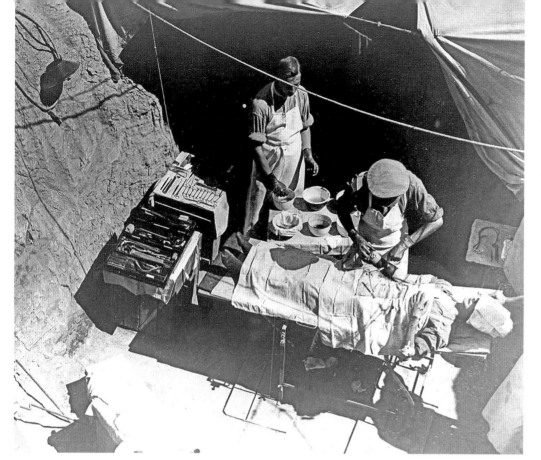

During quiet periods, the resident parson would do his utmost to offer spiritual comfort to those in need, and when they had time, nurses would sit with patients to help them write letters home. They also recorded events and feelings in their own personal diaries. Official daily log entries, however, gave some indication of the continual flow of casualties. A report dated 16 August 1916 at St Johns' hospital stated:

> *Between the 9th and the 15th we received three convoys of wounded, one consisted of four special stretcher cases admitted from No. 15 Ambulance train. These were all of an exceedingly serious nature and one man died an hour and a half after admission. The second convoy arrived at 2.15am on the 11th and numbered seventy-two – all of which were stretcher cases, and as usual composed of most dangerously wounded men. We had some trouble at the pumping station on the 9th and very urgent orders were issued to curtail supply as much as possible.[2]*

The report ends on a reasonably cheery note, stating that the hospital stores had just received 3,000 pairs of socks. Most of these were distributed to the soldiers to prevent trench foot.

Subsequent models of field hospitals and their communities were very similar to those established on the Western Front. They

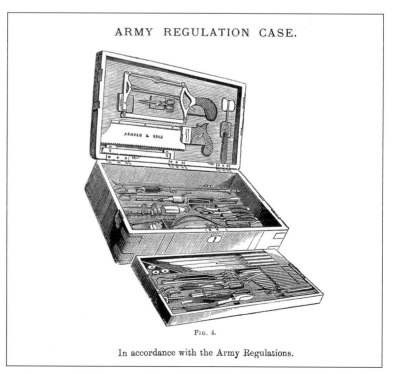

ARMY REGULATION CASE.

ARNOLD & SONS

FIG. 4.

In accordance with the Army Regulations.

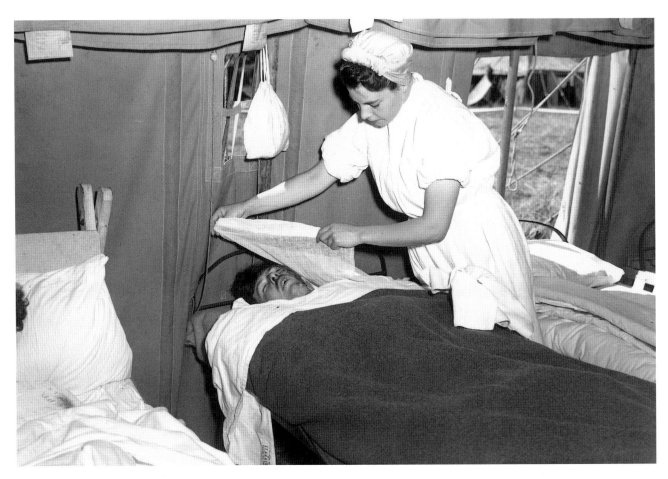

may have varied in size, name, mobility and geographical location but staff efforts to save lives and maintain morale against all odds was undiminished. Everyday irritations such as tea leaves blocking drains, water or supply shortages, electricity problems and staff illnesses paled into insignificance when placed alongside horrendously wounded casualties and high mortality rates. Moreover, despite subsequent and major changes in weaponry, the aetiology of deaths from battlefield wounds has remained remarkably unchanged. Thus, the proportion of deaths from haemorrhage and traumatic head wounds in later conflicts were not dissimilar to those found on the Western Front.

However, during the Second World War soldiers were not confined to trench warfare. Fighting units were far more mobile and covered a wide variety of geographical areas. Therefore, military hospitals were required to be highly mobile and operational within 48 hours. A nurse working for the 75th British General Hospital in Normandy explained the set-up:

Each of us was detailed to a different part. For instance, I was detailed to help unpack resuscitation. You knew that crates belonging to resuscitation were labelled in a certain way. Crates were delivered and you got cracking immediately with claw hammers. Out came the nails and then out came the sacks and then out came the little bundles of oiled instruments. Orderlies came up and put up trestles for stretchers. The boards had to have these collapsible beds fitted out. And then it was all hands to the pump to make up the beds because it was operational in 48 hours. In fact, our first casualties started coming in from Caen and we hadn't found the morphia. We were still diving into the packing case to try and find the morphia. We found it pretty soon because it was necessary, but that's how quickly things happened. It was mostly improvisation inside the tents. We had a trestle as a sort of instruments table, to put out the tray which would hold sterilised syringes, and a small steriliser that was worked by spirit.

ABOVE A British nurse pulls a fly net over an injured soldier at a field hospital near Bayeux in Normandy on 15 August 1944. The region in summer was particularly prone to insects, especially mosquitoes, which made living conditions for servicemen in the field particularly uncomfortable. *(USNA)*

OPPOSITE Sergeant Roger Pouit, French Force, United Nations, helps a wounded North Korean soldier light a cigarette at an aid station, 23rd Regiment, US 2nd Infantry Division. *(IWM MH32970)*

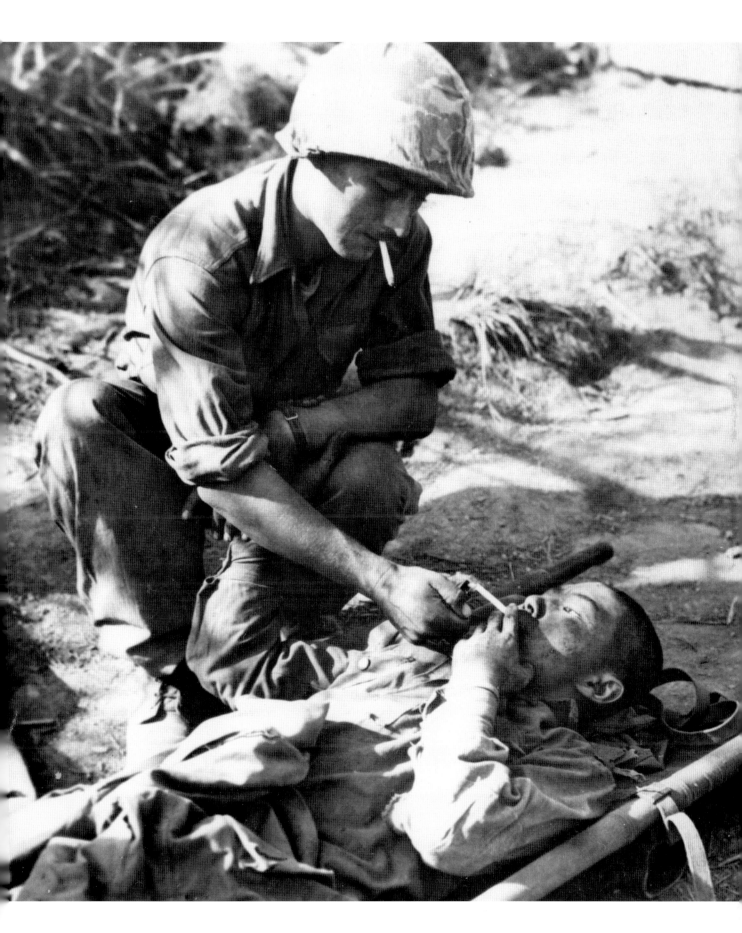

Behind this we stacked compo boxes, as we called them. They were wooden boxes that this compressed tea came in. We stacked them and they acted as shelves for various medicaments, and aspirins, indigestion mixtures, plaster and bandages. We used to have a dustbin for splints, a big blood box somewhere handy and there would be one or two drip stands handy.[3]

Before the outbreak of the Korean War the concept of MASH was already on the drawing board. Based on the two previous global conflicts, MASH evolved to take centre stage in both Korea and Vietnam. There were ten US MASH units situated at various locations in Korea, and a Norwegian MASH (NORMASH). Together these units provided medical support for between 80,000 to 100,000 US and UN forces. Based in tented accommodation with very primitive furniture and equipment, life in MASH was frequently dismal and wretched. Doctors usually slept six to a tent while nurses were grouped in slightly larger accommodation. The five operating tables were often stretchers balanced on carpenters' cutting frames, and food, medicines, intravenous fluids and toiletries were often in short supply. Bed capacity expanded rapidly from 60 to 200 beds, but basic triage was often conducted outside the main tents with stretchers spread out across the ground. Crucially, there were suitable landing sites for MEDEVAC helicopters nearby, which were aided in their work by US and Allied air supremacy.

For field hospital staff, there were lengthy periods of inactivity and boredom, interspersed with frantically busy spells, initiated by piles of incoming wounded. During hectic periods doctors, anaesthetists, nurses and orderlies would work flat out, sometimes not sleeping properly for weeks at a time. MASH units, despite their limited bed capacity, could receive anywhere between 300 and 500 patients in one night. Injuries mainly consisted of extremity, brain and abdominal wounds. When they were not receiving battle casualties, more mundane medical conditions dominated day-to-day life. Summers were characterised by heat exhaustion, dehydration and dermatitis, while the winters brought frostbite and hypothermia to the hospital tents. MASH units were designed to move roughly once a month and basic facilities were augmented by 'add-on' medical support such as laboratories, pharmacies and X-ray departments. Separate tents were also set aside for kitchen, dining and administrative tasks. As in earlier conflicts there were various efforts to shore up staff and patient morale. Cinema screenings, musical concerts, book swapping, outdoor games and gymnastics all played a part in lifting spirits and building a cohesive medical team. US Army officials also enlisted local interpreters to assist with both medical and military intelligence gathering.

Compared to other field hospitals, MASH were highly mobile, but they still required at least 50 trucks to transport them to new locations and took 24 hours to construct. Senior officials would order medical staff to prepare for a move six hours before trucks arrived, but road links were frequently inadequate and massive casualty loads sometimes delayed relocations. One MASH unit (8228th) became a designated haemorrhagic fever hospital, which precluded staff from accepting other casualties. But aside from this medical facility MASH units essentially provided care along the lines of British casualty clearing stations. The quality of US medical supplies, however, was often not up to scratch. Lieutenant Colonel J. Watts, Royal Army Medical Corps, explained:

Plaster of Paris technique, was, on the whole, poor, the plaster bandages used lacked the strength of the Gypsona bandages used in British medical units and plasters were often unduly thick, in consequence. Plastergrams (drawing of the wound on the plaster) with added notes and date, were conspicuous by their absence and the thick plaster, although split, often tended to compress the limb and it was felt that it would be safer to bivalve them and maintain the position with bandages.[4]

Wounds sustained early in the war were due to high-velocity bullets and hand grenades; later in the conflict shellfire and mines caused most damage. A British Field Surgical Team was attached to MASH from October 1950 to March 1951 and Commonwealth surgeons gave

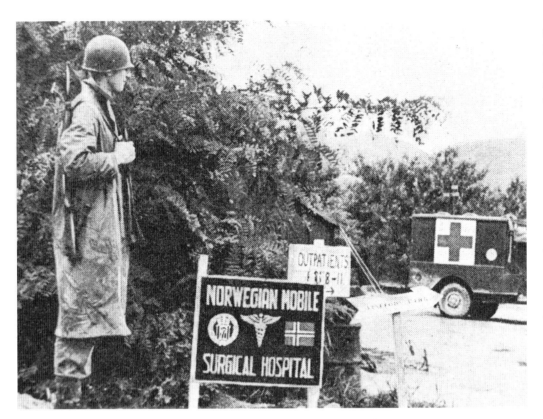

support to the NORMASH. All Commonwealth casualties, except for those requiring neurosurgery, were eventually cared for at the Commonwealth General Hospital in Kure, Japan. Neurosurgical cases were transported to a specialised US centre in Tokyo. In the early stages of care, casualties were given analgesia, immediate first aid, prophylactic penicillin and booster anti-tetanus injections. Delayed primary suture of wounds was favoured, and new treatments for skin grafting were introduced in circumstances where this was not an option. As Lieutenant Colonel Watts recalled:

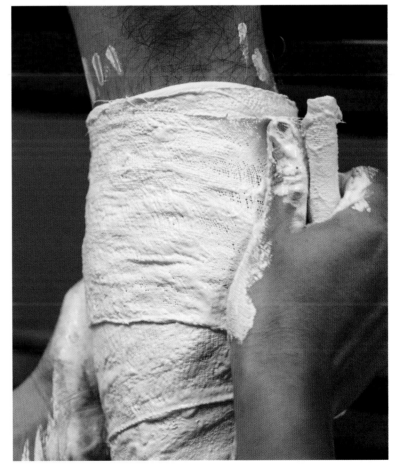

The grafting of massive buttock wounds presents difficulties in dressing the graft so that it does not become detached or soiled, and this led to Lt. Col. E.S.R. Hughes of the Royal Australian Army Medical Corps, who was the senior Australian surgeon at the time, to try a procedure of leaving postage stamp grafts exposed to the air, without dressings and then nursing the patient prone. This resulted in a most successful 'take' and the method was later extended to all areas where it could be used, with extremely satisfying results, even in the

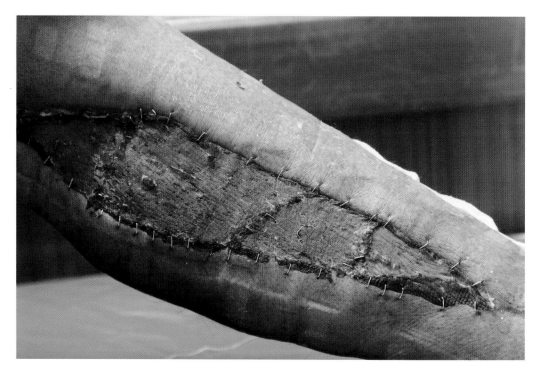

presence of pyocyaneus infection a 50 to 60 per cent take was recorded.[5]

Watts was further impressed by vascular surgery advances in field hospitals, especially the successful vein grafts, which were used to replace severed arteries. He was also pleased with certain war surgery equipment provided in base hospitals, such as Stryker beds for nursing paraplegic patients, electric cast cutters for speedily relieving patients of their plaster of Paris and electric dermatone instruments, used to cut split skin grafts. He was later thrilled to acquire his own electrical plaster cutter, from the Atom Bomb Casualty Commission and a Stryker-type bed frame, which was enthusiastically constructed by the Royal Australian Electrical and Mechanical Engineers. Sadly, he could not afford the $264 required to purchase an electric dermatone.

Acknowledging that medical care in Korea had been somewhat lax at the beginning of the conflict, Watts nevertheless commended base hospitals for 'the excellence of the forward documentation, the notes of the cases were clear, concise and informative, and materially assisted in the handling at base hospitals'. One gem, not be taken as an example, read as follows: 'Ischio-rectal abscess, acute, severe recurrent (I think this guy is nuttier than a fruit cake). Treatment: Wet packs, penicillin. Disposal: To UK facilities Japan. P.S. – Be sure you look at all his tattoos, Jeepers Crow, what a knuckle head.'[6]

Improvements in vascular surgery and skin grafting continued to be a feature of later conflicts. Although many of the field hospitals in Vietnam began as mobile units and assumed fixed roles as the war progressed, expandable sections containing radiology, pharmacy, neurology, laboratory and dental departments were added on as and when necessary. Vietnamese guerrilla warfare tactics encouraged the proliferation of MEDEVAC helicopters, and medical units, self-contained, transportable surgical hospitals (MUST) emerged to help take the strain. Injury patterns varied considerably from those sustained in Korea. Between October 1966 and July 1967, the second MASH unit to be active in Vietnam performed surgery on 1,011 cases. These consisted of high-velocity wounds, vascular trauma, colorectal and burn injuries. Exploratory laparotomies were performed more frequently because abdominal injuries were not always obvious. Ordinary burns were treated with sulfamylon and phosphorous burns received aggressive debridement.[7]

An increasing number of soldiers in Vietnam also suffered from acute respiratory distress syndrome (ARDS). Known colloquially as 'Da Nang Lung', these casualties required ventilation with continuous positive airway pressure in order to maintain correct levels of arterial oxygenation. The value of this new treatment was demonstrated by Colonel Hardaway and Dr Ashbaugh, and resulted in substantial improvements in ventilator management. This in turn contributed to advances in critical care nursing. Better fluid resuscitation reduced mortality rates by 50% and the insertion of central venous lines guided fluid-replacement protocols. Efficient manometer monitors were introduced to measure central venous pressure, blood gases were obtained via arterial catheter and cumbersome glass blood bottles were replaced with lighter plastic containers.[8]

In a conflict that lasted decades, medical care in Vietnam field hospitals evolved slowly and surely to incorporate new methods of fracture fixations and amputations, advances in reconstructive orthoplastic hand surgery and innovations in vascular treatments. In 1962 the US Army established a blood programme to encourage the use of fresh whole blood in forward medical facilities, primarily because of the hepatitis risk associated with other blood products at this time. Blood was distributed from the 406th medical laboratory in Japan, with the walking blood bank making up for any shortfall. Anti-coagulants such as heparin were used with good effect, and the introduction of flying intensive care units ensured continuous resuscitation for the wounded. One of the pioneers in venous repair surgery and Chief of Surgery at 2nd surgical hospital Lai Khe, Major Norman Rich, compiled a Vietnam Vascular Registry, which contained detailed surgical records of 7,500 men. These proved to be invaluable for reference and research purposes.

Dealing with wounded and sick personnel in a tropical climate was not easy. As the war progressed the number of hospital admissions suffering from non-battle medical conditions gradually usurped combat injuries. Between 1965 and 1969 two-thirds of field hospital admissions were due to malaria, hepatitis, diarrhoea, skin infections, fevers of unknown origin and meningococcal meningitis. Infection control measures were introduced, and head and bed nets were supplied to keep

mosquitoes at bay. Repellents were used liberally on the skin and personnel instructed to wear long sleeves. Chloroquine medication was routinely administered to those in the field and about to be deployed, and more laboratory facilities were ushered into field hospitals. But the first case of chloroquine-resistant plasmodium falciparum malaria had already been reported in 1959, necessitating the use of pyrimethamine-dapsone. Resistance to chloroquine remained a severe problem and malaria continued to cause illness and death among US troops. This situation prompted extensive research programmes and scientists at the US Walter Reed Army Medical Centre

BELOW Map of US MASH Units in Vietnam – locations of major medical treatment facilities in Vietnam by the end of 1968. *(Adapted from the Medical Support of the US Army in Vietnam: US Army Office of Medical History)*

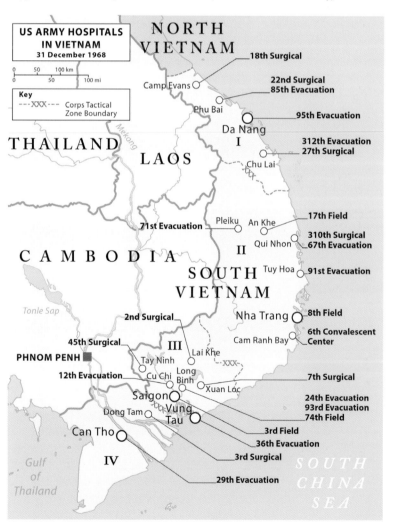

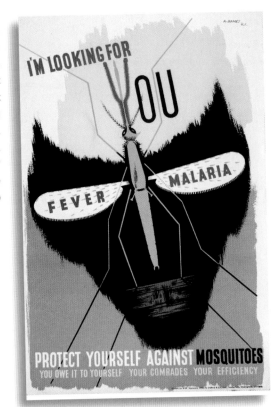

I'M LOOKING FOR YOU

FEVER MALARIA

PROTECT YOURSELF AGAINST MOSQUITOES
YOU OWE IT TO YOURSELF YOUR COMRADES YOUR EFFICIENCY

urgently worked on developing effective anti-malarial strategies. Their research eventually led to discovery of mefloquine. Effective vaccines against meningococcal meningitis also emerged as a result of military research.

In addition to treating war wounded and tropical diseases, field medics were also required to care for an increasing number of psychiatric cases. Clearly, serving in a conflict where both the front line and the enemy was largely invisible took its toll on troop morale and levels of individual sanity. Booby-trapped mines, unpredictable ambushes and other guerrilla tactics produced a 'war of nerves'. Psychiatrists were working in combat zones, but many were overwhelmed by the prevalence and degree of psychosis. A proportion of soldiers developed psychiatric symptoms as a result of adverse reactions to chloroquine, others from combat exhaustion or severe dehydration. But easy and affordable access to mind-altering recreational drugs added to psychiatric diagnostic dilemmas. In response to the latter problem Major M. Grossman, Chief of Medical Staff at 85th evacuation hospital in Phu Bai, established a drug treatment and rehabilitation centre in 1970.

Other problems hindering work in the field hospitals included: plagues of frogs, infestations of lice and leeches, venomous snakes washed up during the monsoon season and interrupted water and electrical supplies. Thus, it was not uncommon for hospital staff to live in damp, squalid conditions and perform surgery by torchlight.

Medical facilities frequently came under serious enemy fire, since the red cross symbol had no meaning in guerrilla warfare. The 45th surgical hospital in Tay Ninh, for example, was obliterated by hostile bombing in November 1966, killing its Commanding Officer Major G. Wratten. Within a matter of days hospital staff and equipment were relocated to the east of Tay Ninh but came under fire again. This led some medics to speculate that red cross insignia merely served as a focus for enemy target practice.

Medics were trained to take cover and appropriate evasive action when under fire, but this was not always possible. Others experienced nerve-racking threats of a more sinister nature, such as the presence of unexploded bombs embedded in field hospital buildings. During the Falklands Campaign, Dr Rick Jolly established a field hospital near a communications satellite in a disused refrigeration plant at Ajax Bay. When 40 Commando came under aerial bombardment in the San Carlos area in May 1982, medics quickly moved into action to save the ensuing casualties. During the general mayhem an RAF Flight Lieutenant called Alan Swan, a bomb disposal expert who was lodging at Ajax Bay, discovered a big problem, as Jolly recounted:

He came up to me and said quietly: 'Excuse me Sir – but will you come and look at this please?' He took me back to one of the refrigeration spaces, two walls away from where the surgical teams were in action. The lights were out, but the strong beam of his torch picked out an incredible sight. Embedded in the grey metal pipework of the refrigeration machinery at the far end of the compartment was a greenish metal cylinder. From one end, a tangled skein of nylon webbing led up to what looked like a parachute, half-pulled through a neat hole behind it. When Alan told me this was a French 400kg high-explosive bomb my first instinct was to turn and run. He grinned at my evident discomfort, and then told me of a second device, lying on the other side of a bulge in the ceiling just above our heads![9]

Jolly was further dismayed to discover that one of the French devices had a time-delay fuse that could last anything up to 37 hours. Since the ground surrounding the refrigeration plant was unsuitable for tented accommodation, and with an advance of Goose Green scheduled for the following day, a tactical decision was made to reinforce the ceiling and protect adjacent walls with sandbags to absorb any subsequent blast. The immediate area was evacuated and cordoned off, but medical work in the remaining section of the field hospital continued as normal. Jolly recalled: 'Instinct swayed my final decision. I thought it highly unlikely that if the first bomb in the stick of four had an impact fuze which

BELOW Disused refrigeration plant at Ajax Bay, used by the British as a field hospital during the Falklands Campaign. *(IWM FKD93)*

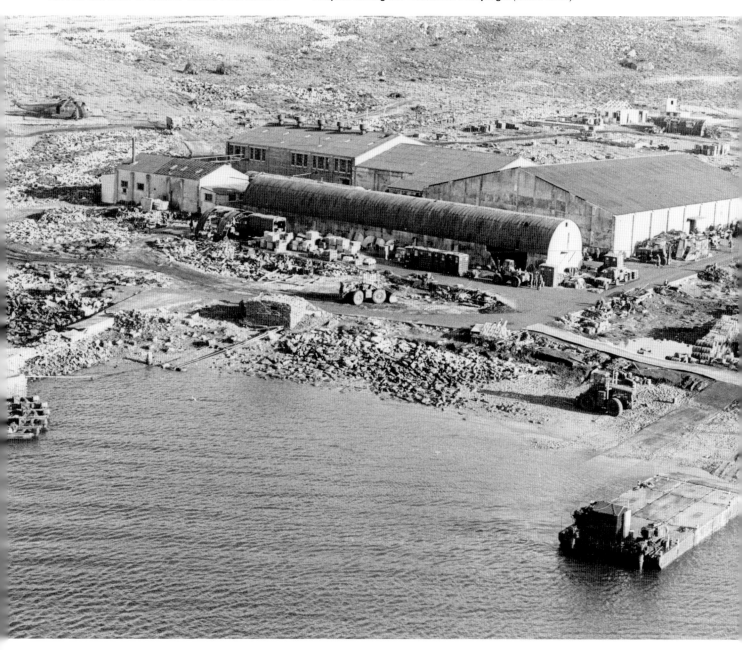

seemed to have detonated successfully that the remainder would have been fitted with time devices instead. This one must have had an impact fuze that had failed.'[10]

Following discussions with his senior medical staff, Jolly moved operating tables closer to the main exit and reduced existing hospital space by 50%, though he omitted to inform them of the prospect of time-delay bomb detonation and the precautions taken to mitigate against such a disaster. At the end of the 37-hour period, however, he handed out tots of rum to all staff members. Nicknamed the 'Red and Green Life Machine' after the beret colours of the British Royal Marines and the Parachute Regiment, the field hospital at Ajax Bay became a beacon of hope for more than 1,000 combat casualties, from both sides of the conflict. As the British advanced eastwards, Jolly also formed additional medical aid facilities at Teal Inlet in the north and Fitzroy in the south. Moreover, when taking care of Argentinian combatants, it quickly became obvious to British surgical teams that Argentinian surgeons had no experience of war surgery.

Bullet wounds, for instance, send shock waves through the body which rapidly create a cavity drawing contaminants into the wound track. Capillary networks then become overly stretched and rupture as a result, causing profuse bleeding into the wound area. This disrupts oxygen supply to muscles and surrounding tissue, exacerbating the risk of infection. Yet Argentinian surgeons seemed to be unaware of the special considerations required to deal with any form of ballistic injury. As Jolly explained:

Real complication occurs when dying muscle tissue is also infiltrated with bacteria or bugs that can cause gas gangrene and tetanus. These are anaerobic in their nature – germs that simply love the absence of oxygen. Any surgeon foolish enough (or emotionally upset and unable to remember the training) who tidies up the entrance and exit holes, then closes the wound off with clips or stitches, was simply asking for trouble. Infection would be inevitable and was present in all our Argentine patients who had been treated

BELOW The Falkland Islands. (Shutterstock)

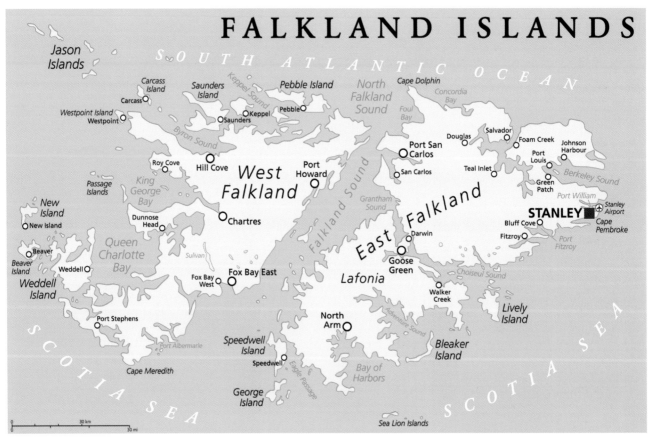

by their own doctors in the field. Some idiot of a mendicant barber surgeon on their side was putting clips in the wounds and giving his patients a few antibiotic tablets. But how was this blood-borne penicillin supposed to penetrate into a load of dead muscle tissue that had no circulation? Their small-arms wounds were much the same, because both sides were using derivatives of the same FN [FN Herstal] rifle design, which fires a 7.62mm round. What was different was the way that our surgeons, with war experience that the Argentine doctors lacked, got on and tackled these wounds. We laid them open to the air then carefully removed the dark purple bits of dead tissue. The work was careful and thorough, demanding intense concentration and a sharp pair of scissors.[11]

Rick Jolly was later awarded the Order of the British Empire by Queen Elizabeth II, and the Orden de Mayo of Argentina for his extraordinary, life-saving work in caring for both British and enemy soldiers in the Falklands.

Taking care of the enemy was nothing new, however; in previous conflicts medics had patched up hostile troops in much the same way as Jolly and his surgical teams had at Ajax Bay. But there were substantial risks to this humanitarian approach. Enemy forces in Korea and Vietnam were not averse to wiring themselves to explosives before entering a hospital for treatment, and then detonating them as soon as they were through the front door. This problem resurfaced in Iraq and Afghanistan with the emergence of suicide bombers. Changes in war conditions and controversy over medical support issues compounded the situation because more civilians began seeking medical attention. With Operation Desert Storm, over 50,000 US troops were deployed along with thousands of coalition forces. Medical assets were mobilised to support rapidly advancing military units and larger CSHs were introduced to work in tandem with mobile MASH facilities. Generally, CSHs could hold up to 200 patients, and provided an efficient intensive-care capability along with four operating tables. Deployable medical systems

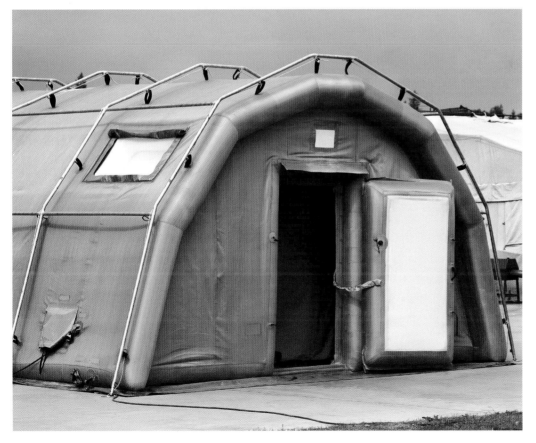

LEFT This field hospital utilises a structure based on inflatable framed modular sections. Its size can be varied depending on requirements and it can be used as a permanent (several years) or temporary (few weeks) facility. *(Shutterstock)*

(DEPMEDS) were attached to CSHs and sent to forward areas as required. Smaller groups of medics, created to move ahead of MASH units, also formed FSTs. These consisted of a triage section, two operating tables and six critical care beds. The latter group could be operational within 2 hours but only contained enough medical supplies for 36 hours.

In the aftermath of Desert Storm there was a review of medical support facilities. US Army officials were beginning to doubt the forward capabilities of MASH – arguing that such units were too slow for modern warfare. Although writing in 2004, a US medic serving in Iraq pointed out:

The most pressing difficulties arise from the changing conditions of the war. Medical teams were designed and outfitted for lightning-quick, highly mobile military operations. The war, however, has proved to be slow-moving and protracted. To adapt, combat support hospitals have had to be converted into fixed facilities. In Baghdad, for example, the 28th CSH took over and moved into an Iraqi hospital in the green zone. This shift has brought increasing numbers of civilians seeking care, and there is no overall policy about providing it. Some hospitals refuse to treat civilians for fear that some may be concealing bombs. Others are treating Iraqis but find themselves overwhelmed, particularly by paediatric patients, for whom they have limited personnel and few supplies.[12]

Clearly the process of treating large numbers of civilian and/or hostile forces also detracted from the main aim of the field hospital, that of providing combat medical support. Doubts about the capabilities of MASH were also unfounded. The 212th MASH, for example, successfully provided medical support to advancing troops, with surgeons performing 100 operations between 27 March and 14 April 2003. With 36 beds, 2 operating tables and 6 resuscitation beds, this field hospital played a crucial role in Operation Iraqi Freedom. Construction time had also been reduced from 24 to 12 hours. Despite this considerable success, the days of MASH were numbered, and the last unit was decommissioned in 2006.

A combination of CSHs and FSTs had largely taken over the role of MASH before this date. The demise of the latter was hastened in part by the need to provide more FSTs, but also by new and revolutionary attitudes to battlefield medicine. By the mid-1990s ideas of damage-control resuscitation and damage-control surgery had replaced older, more traditional approaches to casualty care.

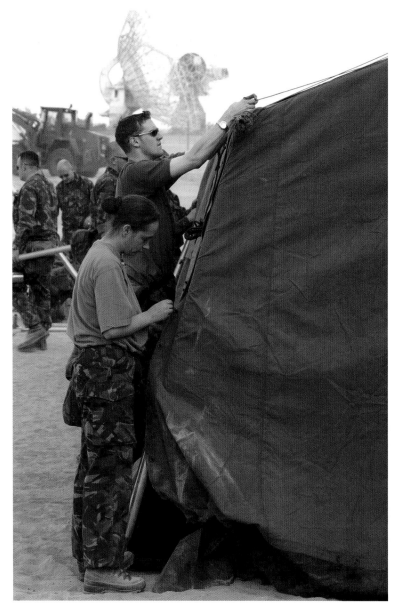

BELOW Members of 33 Field Hospital of the RAMC arrive in Kuwait and put up a tented hospital, which will form part of the mobile hospital.
(IWM OP-TELIC 03-010-08-001)

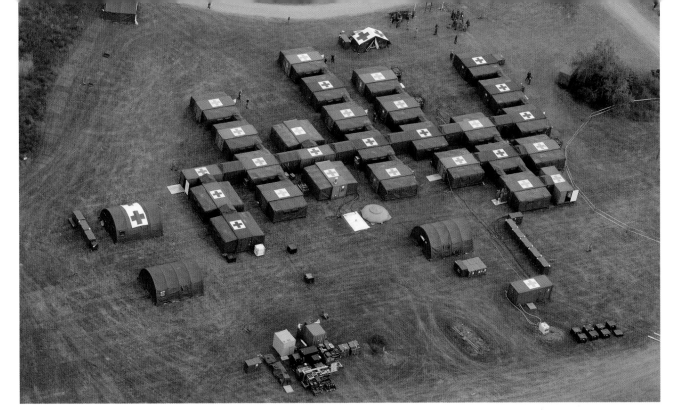

Henceforth, by including trauma specialists and anaesthetists in forward surgical and MERT, highly skilled resuscitation and emergency care could be provided at the scene of wounding, on a par with that initially administered in hospital emergency departments. Damage control required combat medics to do only what was necessary to save life and limb in the first instance and delay definitive repair until a later stage. Other trauma innovations included consultant-led care, standardised training programmes and treatment guidelines, real-time system evaluation and enhancement, rehabilitation to achieve occupation reintegration and effective clinical and scientific research.[13] Military diagnostics was also improved by advances in digital technology, CT, ultrasound equipment with internet connections to specialist consultants and electronic data transfer.

Greater integration of NATO medical forces also improved casualty care. A research study which examined patient outcomes in a multinational Role-three combat hospital in Kandahar revealed that between 1 October 2009 and 31 December 2010 medics treated a large volume of severely injured patients. However, mortality rates were exceptionally low – 4.45%. By consolidating specialities in a high-volume centre, this multinational facility achieved superlative outcomes.[14] Other Role-three field

hospitals, such as that led by the UK at Camp Bastion, echoed this success.

Furthermore, the unparalleled dedication of combat medics had not wavered over the course of a century. Within the trauma bays and operating theatres of Camp Bastion, the critically injured received the same focused, highly skilled, devoted medical attention that was afforded to their ancestors on the Western Front. Mortality rates have plummeted because of life-saving medical advances, but the intensity of battlefield trauma remains the same. Bastion hospital, equipped with sonography and multi-slice computed tomography was clearly laid out, with trauma bays situated left of the entrance and operating theatres to the right; the seriousness of casualties was indicated by a sharp instruction to 'right turn' on arrival. At 5.00pm one evening a junior trauma surgeon received a nine-liner:

[f]our serious casualties, two of them very bad indeed, and they'd waited 30 minutes before it was safe for the MERT to land and collect them. Too long. With one already dead, MERT crew turned away to work on the other, still very bad when unloaded. Right turn at Bastion, everyone there pushing forward to surround where he lay, no heart beat so the junior surgeon opened his chest and reached for the heart itself, massaging it

ABOVE An aerial view of a Role 2 Enhanced field hospital during Exercise Collaborative CanUK at Canadian Forces Base, Kingston, Ontario, in 2015. Role 2 Enhanced provides triage, resuscitation, emergency surgery and essential post-operative management.
(Canadian Forces)

hand to heart, no ribs or chest in between, no muttered song for rhythm, just thin sterile gloves gleaming with blood on a pair of hands and the muscle itself, lying between them, not moving, not responding. Keep going. Blood and adrenaline in through the lines to help him, and finally, after four minutes, the surgeon felt a flutter between his hands, and then a twist and then a rhythm, and he could actually see it moving in the middle of all that blood, beating on, and then – not that he needed it – the monitor bipped a confirmation. No more time to listen, as there were many more injuries,

but now the veins that held the lines were shutting down, so blood must be leaking out somewhere, blood pressure falling, patient falling back, so the team went back after him. His leg was gone, so an amputation to remove what remained just below the knee was being done. Lacerations to the lung, but not serious. Where else? Open up the stomach – blood so dark and deep – a huge haemorrhage, still bleeding, unstoppable, but they tried, more blood in the lines, back and forth, heart massage, but this time no fluttering, no movement, and the team leader called a halt.[15]

BELOW The Medical Treatment Facility (MTF), which is housed in one of the few solid buildings at Bastion, replaces the tented field hospital that had been used since 2003. The temperature-controlled building allows medics to better avoid the heat, cold and dust that come with the Helmand territory. With a fully equipped operating theatre supporting two operating tables, the MTF also supports up to six beds for the most critically injured in an Intensive Treatment Unit (ITU). Two general wards handle patients with recovery needs and there are an additional two separate, private rooms, supplying a total capacity of 37 beds, with room for expansion.
(MOD Open Government Licence)

Bastion field hospital had started out in tented accommodation near an airbase, but slowly evolved; first into pre-fabricated buildings and then into a heavily guarded concrete encampment. A highly capable medical facility, it was able to provide resuscitation, damage-control surgery and intensive care. Staffed by a UK-led multinational team, who had completed 18 months of pre-deployment training following UK clinical Guidelines for Operations, the hospital provided the most advanced in-theatre

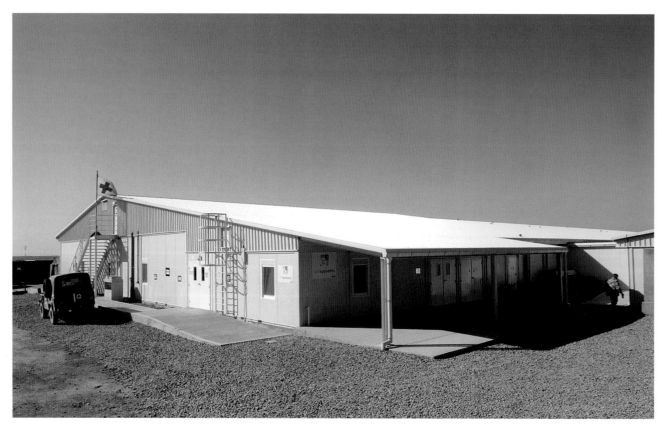

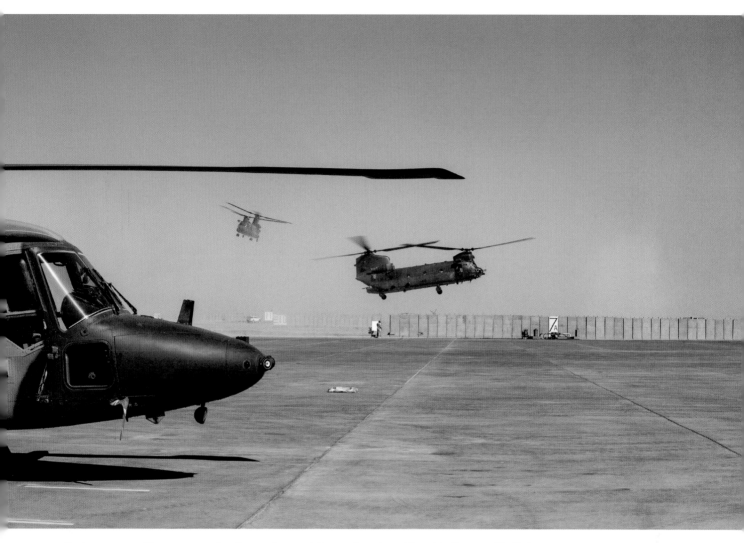

medical resources. The average stay for service personnel was 24 hours, after which UK casualties were airlifted to the Defence Medical Services in Birmingham by CCAST. Referred to as the medical equivalent of a Formula 1 pit stop by one military doctor, a remarkable 98% of casualties admitted through Bastion's doors survived. Elite multinational teams of surgeons, anaesthetists, nurses and radiologists worked with complex, innovative equipment such as 3D imaging, to provide the very best of consultant-led field hospital care. Live link-ups with medics in Birmingham ensured this continuity of medical provision on the home front.

In addition to combat casualties, Bastion hospital received a large cohort of Afghan patients, many of whom needed weeks of care. Interpreters were employed to assist with language, cultural and religious issues, and, just as in Korea and subsequent conflicts, as

interrogators for military intelligence. Similarly, in leisure times, medical staff responded to field hospital life in much the same way as their predecessors. Nurses wrote lengthy cathartic diaries, some for personal use, others designed to be interactive with their patients, detailing their individual medical journeys. The latter were shared with patients and given to them on discharge from hospital to help them come to terms with their critical injuries and chart their future progress and rehabilitation. Other staff, meanwhile, established basic outdoor sports facilities and small gardens within the compound surrounding the hospital. Places for relaxation and solace for rest and reflection, creating an oasis of normality and cultivating nature just as generations of war surgeons had done before. Diaries and gardens, symbols of enduring hope and life amid the atrocities of war.

ABOVE RAF Chinook helicopters come in to land at Camp Bastion. *(Shutterstock)*

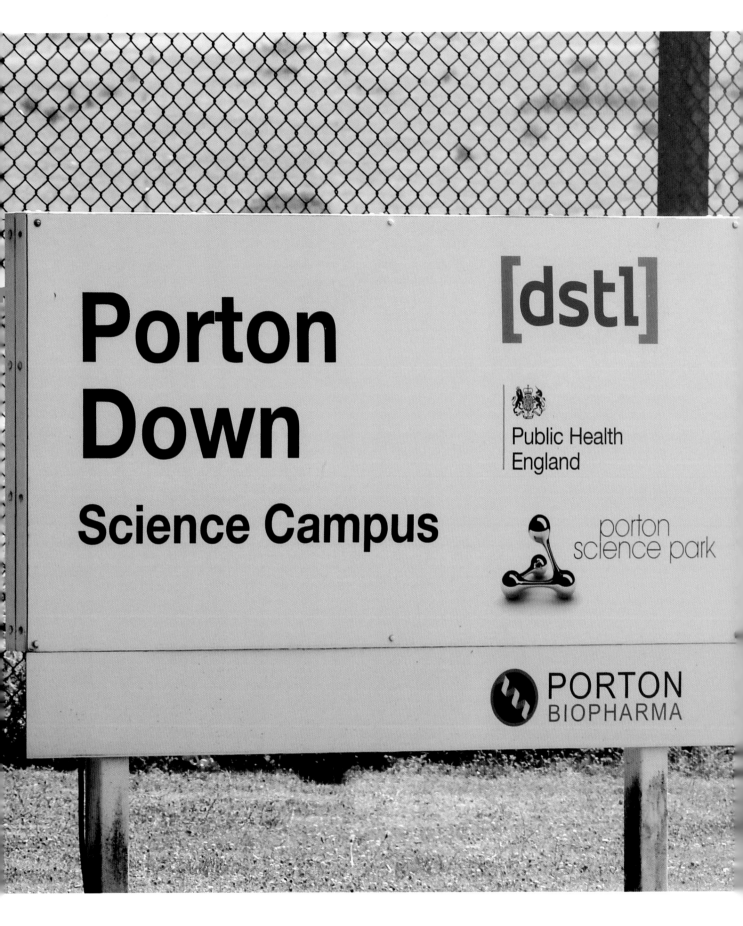

Epilogue

Thanks to innovations in pre-hospital care, evacuation procedures, damage-control resuscitation and damage-control surgery, more UK, US and coalition force casualties have survived recent conflicts. Many of these battle trauma survivors, however, have suffered severe and disabling injuries. Rehabilitation is often a long and laborious process, patiently guided by medical expertise and research. Indeed, the amalgamation of bio-engineering, robotics and neurosurgery have combined to offer new hope to injured military veterans. Furthermore, clinically driven pioneering work at the Royal British Legion Centre for Blast Injury Studies, Imperial College London, is aimed at significantly improving the lives of those already injured and developing optimal military medical strategies for future casualty care. Research is focused on understanding the mechanism and pathophysiology of blast injuries, including musculoskeletal and extremity injuries, heterotopic ossification, hearing loss, TBI, causes of death and next-level survivors and torso trauma.[1]

As Brigadier Tim Hodgetts CBE, Medical Director of the UK Defence Medical Services, has stated:

The Centre is one of the principal academic institutes engaged in medical research in the UK . . . [it] has a critical role to play in the continued knowledge development of blast injuries and will continue to play a major role in delivering valuable research to meet defence medical requirements.[2]

The UK Defence Science and Technology Laboratory at Porton Down is also crucial in terms of medical research. For example, scientists at this establishment were the first to discover that certain blood products, given in pre-hospital care settings, improved survival rates by increasing blood-clotting times in casualties suffering from haemorrhage. They continue to develop pre-treatments and antidotes for use in the event of nerve agent attacks, specific substances to counteract biological threats and clothing to protect military personnel from CBRN attacks. In addition, the Combat Casualty Care Group at Porton Down continually analyse emerging injury patterns from the battlefield; they then identify and prioritise research areas. The results of these investigations are subsequently circulated to senior military officials to improve pre-deployment medical training and battlefield preparation.

Extensive scientific research and clinical facilities are available to all UK military services. Much of the current work is multidisciplinary and involves collaboration with the USA and other NATO members. Some of these investigations and analytical processes are force-specific. One thing is certain, however: combat medicine will continue to rely on the expertise of highly trained military medics, and evolve in response to changing methods of warfare and the dissemination of medical research findings.

OPPOSITE The Defence Science and Technology Laboratory at Porton Down near Salisbury, in the West of England. *(Shutterstock)*

BELOW Help for Heroes is a British charity launched in 2007 to help provide better facilities for British servicemen and women who have been wounded or injured in the line of duty. *(Shutterstock)*

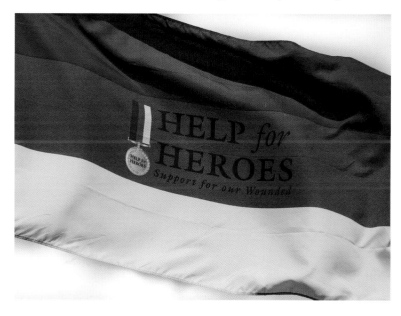

Endnotes

Chapter 1

1. P. Starns, *Sisters of the Somme* (Stroud: The History Press, 2016), p. 91.
2. NATO Logistics Handbook Medical Support, 1997.
3. National Archive WO/222/23.
4. Ibid.
5. F. Omori, *Quiet Heroes: Navy Nurses of the Korean War 1950–1953* (St Paul, MN: Smith House Press, 2000), p. 90.
6. Captain Jane Titley ARRC, Matron-in-Chief Queen Alexandra's Royal Naval Nursing Service 1991–94, interview with author, June 1994.
7. NATO Logistics Handbook Medical Operational Principles, 2016.
8. C. Benjamin and M. McCarten, 'Saving Lives in the Heat of Battle' (2011), p. 1. Available at: https://www.hsph.harvard.edu/news/magazine/alumni-military-medicine.
9. Squadron Leader Garth Logan, SO2 Aeromed Aeromedical Evacuation Control Centre, RAF Tactical Medical Wing. Email correspondence with author, 12 December 2018.
10. NATO Logistics Handbook – article 1605, k., 'Listed Medical Operational Principles', 1997.
11. L. Hourani, C. Council, R. Hubal and L. Strange, 'Approaches to the Primary Prevention of Post-Traumatic Stress Disorder in the Military: A Review of Stress Control Literature', *Journal of Military Medicine*, 176 (7) (2011), 721–30. See also study funded by US Department of Defense under: W81XWH-08-10334 and N000014-08-C-054.
12. Ibid.
13. S.J. Mercer, C.L. Whittle and P.F. Mahoney, 'Lessons from the Battlefield: Human Factors in Defence Anaesthesia', *British Journal of Anaesthesia*, 108 (1) (2010), 9–10.
14. Ibid.
15. Ibid.
16. C. Thompson-Edgar, interview for the *Mail on Sunday*, 1 March 2015.
17. P.S. London, FRCS, 'Medical Lessons for the Falkland Islands Campaign', Report of a Meeting of the United Services Section of the Royal College of Medicine, held at the Royal College of Surgeons 17 and 18 February 1983.
18. J.J. Hodgetts and P.F. Mahoney, 'Redefining the Military Trauma Paradigm', *Journal of Emergency Medicine*: British Association of Accident and Emergency Medicine, 23 (10) (2006), 745–46.
19. US Defense Department Handbook. Details can also be found at www.goarmy.com.

Chapter 2

1. R. Jolly, *Doctor for Friend and Foe* (London: Conway Maritime Press, 2012), pp. 181–82.
2. Ibid., p. 119.
3. US Army, 68W Combat Medical Pocket Guide, 2018.
4. Omori, *Quiet Heroes*, pp. 34–35.
5. Thompson-Edgar, interview for the *Mail on Sunday*, 1 March 2015.
6. T.C. Nicholson Roberts and R.D. Berry, 'Pre-hospital Trauma Care and Aero-medical Transfer: A Military Perspective', *British Journal of Anaesthesia*: Continuing Education in Anaesthesia Critical Care & Pain, 12 (4) (August 2012), 186–89.
7. E. Mayhew, *A Heavy Reckoning: War Medicine and Survival in Afghanistan and Beyond* (London: Profile Books, 2017) p. 25.
8. Ibid.
9. R. Nandra, P. Park and K. Porter, 'From Bastion to Birmingham: What Have We Learnt from Acute Military Trauma and How Has it Impacted on Emergency Treatments of Civilian Trauma?' *Journal of Orthoplastic Surgery*, 1 (September 2018), 26–32.
10. Ibid.
11. Ibid.

Chapter 3

1. National Archive WO/222/189/6.
2. School of Aerospace Medicine, United States Aerospace Medical Centre (ATC), Brooks Air Force Base, Texas. Reference: 264462, Langdon, D., *Air Evacuation of Patients with Head Injuries*, 26 September 1961, p. 5.
3. Ibid.
4. Ibid., p. 9.
5. Omori, *Quiet Heroes*, p. 100.
6. US Navy Bureau of Medicine and Surgery Archives: *Life and Health* magazine, 'The Ship with a Heart', July 1952.
7. Omori, *Quiet Heroes*, p. 132.
8. M. Novosel, 'Medical Memoirs 1969–1970', AMEDD Medical History. See also M. Novosel, *Dust Off: Memoirs of an Army Aviator* (Novatio, CA: Presidio, 1999).
9. Ibid.
10. Jolly, *Doctor for Friend and Foe*, pp. 114–15.

11. See: https://www.airforcemedicine.af.mil/News/Display/Article/1466825/the-evolution-of-aeromedical-evacuation-capabilities-help-deployed-medicine-take-flight.
12. A. Gawande, 'Casualties of War – Military Care for the Wounded from Iraq and Afghanistan', *New England Journal of Medicine*, 351 (24) (9 December 2004), 2471–75.
13. Flight Sergeant Kevin Swift talking to BBC Television News TV news correspondent L. Wilkins, 9 June 2011.
14. Wing Commander Robert Tipping, MB BS DAvMED FRCA SO1 Aviation Medicine Consultant Adviser in Pre-Hospital Care to Hd RAFMS. Email correspondence with author, 30 January 2019.
15. Squadron Leader Garth Logan. Email correspondence with author, 12 December 2018.
16. Wing Commander Robert Tipping, MB BS DAvMED FRCA SO1 Aviation Medicine Consultant Adviser in Pre-Hospital Care to Hd RAFMS. Email correspondence with author, 30th January 2019.
17. Ibid.
18. Squadron Leader Garth Logan. Email correspondence with author, 12 December 2018.
19. Wing Commander Peter D. Hodkinson, Consultant in Aviation and Space Medicine, RAF Centre of Aviation Medicine. Email correspondence with author, 14 December 2018.
20. Wing Commander Robert Linfield, 'RAF 400M Atlas to Be Used for Medevac', 28 May 2018. See: https://www.airmedandrescue.com/storyhttps://www.airmedrescue.com for further information.

Chapter 4

1. R.D. Dripps, 'Anaesthesia for Combat Casualties on the Basis of Experience in Korea'. Paper presented to the Army Medical Service Graduate School, Walter Reed US Army Medical Centre, Washington, DC, 19 April 1954, published in: *Medical Science Publication*, 4 (1) pp. 117–131.
2. Colonel J.A. Jenicek MC (Ret), 'The New Face of Anaesthesiology in Vietnam', *Journal of Military Medicine* (October 1997).
3. London, 'Medical Lessons from the Falkland Islands Campaign'.
4. Jolly, *Doctor for Friend and Foe*, p. 143.
5. S.J. Mercer, 'Clinical Anaesthesia in the Armed Forces: A History of the Tri-Service Apparatus', *Journal of the Royal Naval Medical Services*, 94 (2) (2008), 74–82.
6. Wing Commander Robert Tipping, email correspondence with author, 30 January 2019. NB: Airtraq is a fibre optic device with guided video intubation, which is a helpful tool in circumstances where blood or swelling obstructs the view of the patient's vocal cords.
7. S. Bibian, 'Closed Loop Total Intravenous Anaesthesia: The Battlefield Anaesthetic of the Future', Congressionally Directed United States Defense and Medical Research Programs, 22 March 2017.

Chapter 5

1. Korea: US Department of Veterans Affairs: Military Service History Korea: www.va.gov/OAA/pocketcard/m-korea.asp.
2. M. Washington, M. Brown, T. Palys, S. Tyner and R. Bowden, 'Clinical Microbiology during the Vietnam War', *Military Medicine*, 174 (11) (November 2009), 1209–14.
3. R.M. Hall, 'Medical Year-End Wrap Up, 1967', San Francisco, California, Office of the Command Surgeon, United States Military Assistance Command, Vietnam, 1968.
4. London, 'Medical Lessons from the Falkland Islands Campaign'.
5. Jolly, *Doctor for Friend and Foe*, pp. 123–24.
6. Gawande, 'Casualties of War'.
7. G.R. Mueller, T.J. Pineda, H.X. Xie, J.S. Teach, A.D. Barofsky, J.R. Schmid and K.W. Gregory, 'A Novel Sponge-Based Wound Stasis Dressing to Treat Lethal Non-compressible Haemorrhage, *Journal of Trauma Acute Care Surgery*, 73 (2 Supplement 1) (2012), S134–39.
8. Wing Commander Robert Tipping. Email correspondence with author, 30 January 2019.
9. Lieutenant Colonel Harvey Pynn MA FRCEM DMCC DTM&H DiplMC DMM RAMC, Consultant in Emergency Medicine and Pre-hospital Emergency Medicine Defence Consultant Adviser in Pre-hospital Emergency Care. Email correspondence with author, 15 January 2019.
10. H. Shakur et al., 'Effects of Tranexamic Acid on Death, Vascular Occlusive Events, and Blood Transfusion in Trauma Patients with Significant Haemorrhage (CRASH-2): A Randomised, Placebo-Controlled Trial', *Lancet*, 376 (9734) (3 July 2010), 23–32.
11. J.J. Morrison, J.J. Dubose, T.E. Rasmussen and M.J. Midwinter, 'Military Application of Tranexamic Acid in Trauma Emergency Resuscitation (MATTERS) Study', *Archives of Surgery*, 147 (2012), 113–39.
12. C. Creighton, et al., 'Trauma Care at a Multinational United Kingdom-Led Role-Three Combat Support Hospital: Resuscitation Outcomes from a Multidisciplinary Approach', *Journal of Military Medicine*, 179 (11) (2014), 1258–62.
13. Ibid.

14. London, 'Medical Lessons Learned from the Falkland Islands Campaign'.
15. H.F. Pidcoke et al., 'Ten-Year Analysis of Transfusion in Operation Iraqi Freedom and Operation Enduring Freedom: Increased Plasma and Platelet Use Correlates with Improved Survival', *Journal of Trauma Acute Care Surgery*, 73 (6 Supplement 5) (2012), S445–S452.

Chapter 6

1. National Archive AIR 58/ 484 & AIR 58/374: Royal Institute of Aviation Medicine, 1 January 1973 to 31 December 1973. Air Crew Equipment Group Report 321. Assessment of visual limitations conducted at BA Corporation, Warton, 24 to 25 October 1973.
2. Omori, *Quiet Heroes*, p. 46.
3. US Department of Veterans Affairs: Military Service History Korea.
4. W. Burkhater, 'Surgery in Vietnam: Orthopaedic Surgery', Washington DC, USA, Office of the Surgeon General Department – Army (1994).
5. L.D. Heaton et al., 'Military Surgical Practices of the United States Army in Vietnam', *Current Problems in Surgery* (November 1966), pp. 1–59.
6. S.J. Mennion, 'Principles of War Surgery', *British Medical Journal*, 330 (7506) (23 June 2005), 1498–1500.
7. J.G. Penn-Barwell et al., 'Severe Open Tibial Fractures in Combat Surgery: Management and Preliminary Outcomes', *The Bone and Joint Journal*, 95B (1) (2013), 101–5.
8. J.G. Penn-Barnwell et al., 'Use of Topical Negative Pressure in British Servicemen with Combat Wounds', *Journal of Eplasty*, 11 (2011), e35.
9. London, 'Medical Lessons Learned from the Falkland Islands Campaign'.
10. Ibid.
11. P.J. Belmont et al., 'Epidemiology of Combat Wounds in Iraqi Operation Enduring Freedom: Orthopaedic Burden of Disease', *Journal of Orthopaedic Surgery Advances*, 19 (1) (2010), 2–7.
12. Gawande, 'Casualties of War', 2471–75.
13. Creighton, et al., 'Trauma Care at a Multinational United Kingdom-Led Role-Three Combat Support Hospital'.
14. Ibid.
15. P. Bates et al., 'Demystifying Damage Control in Musculoskeletal Trauma', *Annals of Orthopaedic Surgery*, 98 (5) (2016), 291–94.
16. D. Farina, speaking at Imperial College London, 23 October 2018. Report by C. Brogan. Imperial College press release.

Chapter 7

1. H. Cushing, *From a Surgeon's Journal* (New York: Little, Brown and Company, 1936), p. 14.
2. National Archive WO/222/189/10.
3. Monica Goulding, BBC Radio 4, *Frontline Females* (April 1998).
4. A.M. Meirowsky, 'Wounds of Dural Sinuses', *Journal of Neurosurgery*, 10 (1953), 496–514.
5. 'Military Medical Advances Resulting from the Conflict in Korea. Part 2: Historic Clinical Accomplishments', *Journal of Military Medicine*, 177 (4) (2012), 430–35.
6. Jolly, *Doctor for Friend and Foe*, p. 119.
7. Ibid., pp. 180, 184.
8. London, 'Medical Lessons from the Falkland Islands Campaign'.
9. Jolly, *Doctor for Friend and Foe*, p. 107.
10. Gawande, 'Casualties of War', 2473.
11. G. Ling and J. Ecklund, 'Traumatic Brain Injury in Modern War', *Current Opinion in Anaesthesiology*, 24 (2), (April 2011), 124–30.
12. J.E. Risdall and D.K. Menon, 'Traumatic Brain Injury', Philosophical Transactions of the Royal Society, London Biological Sciences, 2011, January 27; 366 (1562): (27 January 2011), 241–50, at p. 247, quoted in Mayhew, *A Heavy Reckoning*, p. 273.
13. S. Shively et al., 'Research in Context, Editorial Comment On: Characterisation of Interface Astroglial Scarring in the Human Brain after Blast Exposure: A Post Mortem Case Series', quoted in Mayhew, *A Heavy Reckoning*, p. 272.

Chapter 8

1. Official Government Report of the Committee into 'Shell-Shock' (London, HMSO, 1922).
2. M. Baly, oral history interview with the author, 1997.
3. National Archive WO/222/23.
4. 'Military Medical Advances Resulting from the Conflict in Korea. Part 2'.
5. J.J. Flood, 'Psychiatric Casualties in UK Elements of Korean Force December 1950–November 1951', *Journal of Royal Army Medical Corps*, 100 (1) (January 1954), pp. 40–47.
6. Ibid.
7. National Archive WO281/887, 3 August 1953.
8. American Psychiatric Association, Diagnostic and Statistics Manual of Mental Disorders (Washington DC: American Psychiatric Association, 1952).
9. N.M. Camp, 'Ethical Challenges for the Psychiatrist during the Vietnam Conflict', in F.D. Jones et al. (eds), *Military Psychiatry: Preparing in Peace for War* (Washington DC: Office of the Surgeon General, Borden Institute, 1994), pp. 137–40.
10. R.J. Lifton, *Witness to an Extreme Century: A Memoir* (New York: Free Press, New York 2011), p. 176.
11. E. Mayhew, *A Heavy Reckoning: War, Medicine and Survival in Afghanistan and Beyond*, (2017), p. 287.
12. London, 'Medical Lessons from the Falkland Islands Campaign'.

13. Jolly, *Doctor for Friend and Foe*, p. 120.
14. Ibid., p. 187.
15. Ibid., p. 231.
16. T.C. Smith, 'The US Department of Defense Millennium Cohort Study: Career Span and Beyond, Longitudinal Follow-Up', *Journal of Environmental Medicine*, 51 (10) (October 2009). Naval Health Research Centre Report no. 08-38.
17. Operational Stress Management and Trauma Risk Management (TRiM) Cell, OSM & TRIM Team. Navy Command Headquarters. The Royal Navy Trauma Risk Management Handbook. Available at: http://c69011.r11.cf3.rackcdn.com/ d951c5627eb44b3789e84292d1e2c1fa-0x0.pdf, p. 15. –Rackcdn.comc69011.r11.cf3. rackdn.com/d951c5627eb44b3789e8429e84292d1e2c1fa-OxO.pdf.
18. T. Sotomayor et al., 'Severe Trauma Stress Inoculation Training for Combat Medics Using High-Fidelity Simulation, Interservice–Industry Training', Simulation and Education Conference (I/ITSEC), December 2013.
19. P. Roach, *Citizen Surgeon: A Memoir* (Pennsauken: Book Baby, Pennsauken 2014).
20. Mayhew, *A Heavy Reckoning*, p. 29.

Chapter 9

1. Cushing, *From a Surgeon's Journal*, p. 34.
2. J.M. Stellman and S.D. Stellman, 'Agent Orange during the Vietnam War: The Lingering Issue of its Civilian and Military Health Impact', *American Journal of Public Health*, 108 (6) (June 2018), 726–28.
3. J. Bajgar et al., 'Other Toxic Chemicals as Potential Chemical Warfare Agents', in R. Gupta (ed.), *Handbook of Toxicology of Chemical Warfare Agents* edited by R. Gupta (London: Academic Press, 2015), pp. 337–46. Despite its slightly delayed effects, Dioxin was used to poison President Yushchenko of the Ukraine in 2009.
4. US Central Intelligence Agency, Office of National Estimates: Memorandum for the Director, 'Use of Nuclear Weapons in Vietnam', 18 March 1966.
5. Starns, *Sisters of the Somme*, p. 181.
6. Mustard gas was first used by the Germans during the First World War. The British version of mustard gas was made at Avonmouth near Bristol, and the substance was so lethal that nearly 70% of the workforce involved in its production became severely ill. Seven people died in the factory in as many months because safety precautions were inadequate. As late as 2013, chemical experts from Porton Down were required to examine the site for contamination risks before a new factory could be built on the same site.
7. 'Casualty Management', *Journal of the Royal Army Medical Corps*, 149 (2003), 199–202.
8. Ibid.
9. US Department of Veterans Affairs, Gulf War Unique Health Risks, 2019.
10. US General Accounting Office, 'Chemical and Biological Defence: US Forces Are not Adequately Equipped to Detect all Threats' (Washington DC, US Government Printing Office, 1993). Available at: https://www.gao.gov/products/NSIAD-96-103.
11. NATO Standard (AJP-4.10) Allied Joint Doctrine for Medical Support, Edited B Version 1, with UK Elements, May 2015, NATO Standardization Office (NSO).
12. 'Operations in Chemical, Biological, Radiological and Nuclear Environments', Joint Chiefs of Staff, joint publication 3-11, 29 October 2018. Available at: https://www.jcs.mil/ Portals/36/Documents/Doctrine/pubs/jp3_11.pdf?ver=2018-12-07-091639-697.
13. Ibid.

Chapter 10

1. Starns, *Sisters of the Somme*, p. 23.
2. Ibid., pp. 109–10.
3. Goulding, BBC Radio 4, *Frontline Females*.
4. Lieutenant Colonel J.C. Watts RAMC, 'War Surgery in the Korean Campaign', *Post-graduate Medical Journal*, 30 (1 January 1954), 22–29.
5. Ibid.
6. Ibid.
7. B. King and I. Jatoi, 'The Mobile Army Surgical Hospital: A Military and Surgical Legacy', *Journal of the Medical Association*, 97 (5 May 2005), pp. 648–56.
8. Ibid.
9. Jolly, *Doctor for Friend and Foe*, p. 109.
10. Ibid., p. 111.
11. Ibid., p. 140.
12. Gawande, 'Casualties of War'.
13. S. Hettiaratchy, T.N. Mahoney and T. Hodgetts, 'UK's NHS Trauma Systems: Lessons from Military Experience', *Lancet*, 376 (9736) (2010), 149–51.
14. C. Creighton, C Tubb et al., 'Trauma Care at a Multinational United Kingdom-Led Role Three Combat Hospital'.
15. Mayhew, *A Heavy Reckoning*, p. 81.

Epilogue

1. Royal British Legion Centre for Blast Injury Studies, Imperial College London: https:// www.imperial.ac.uk/blast-injury.
2. Ibid.

Appendix 3

1. Major Clinton Jones, Surgeon Commander Simon J. Mercer RN and Colonel Peter F. Mahoney, 'Shaping Military Training in the Era of Contingency and Revalidation', *Bulletin of the Royal College of Anaesthetists*, 97 (May 2016), 41–43.

Bibliography and sources

Cowdrey, A.E., *MASH versus MASH: The Mobile Army Surgical Hospital* (Washington DC: US Army Centre for Military History, Washington DC, 1985)

Cushing, H., *From a Surgeon's Journal* (New York: Little, Brown and Company, 1936)

'Defence Nurses' Experiences from Iraq and Afghanistan: The Defence Nursing Forum's Oral History Project' (London: Royal College of Nursing, London 2015)

Gabriel, A., *Between Flesh and Steel: A History of Military Medicine from the Middle Ages to Afghanistan* (Washington DC: Potomac Books, Nebraska 2013)

Herman, J.K., *Frozen in Memory: US Medicine in the Korean War* (Book locker.com, 2006)

Horwitz, D.G. (ed.), *We Will not Be Strangers: Korean War Letters between a MASH Surgeon and His Wife* (Urbana and Chicago, IL: University of Illinois Press, Illinois 1997)

Jolly, R., *Doctor for Friend and Foe* (London: Conway Maritime Press, London 2012)

Jolly, R., *The Red and Green Life Machine: A Diary of the Falklands Field Hospital* (London: Corgi Press, London 1984)

Jones, E., *Shell Shock to PTSD: Military Psychiatry from 1900 to the Gulf War* (London: Psychology Press, London 2005)

Lifton, R.J., *Witness to an Extreme Century: A Memoir* (New York: Free Press, 2011)

Madison, C., *The War Came Home with Him: A Daughter's Memoir* (Minneapolis, MN: University of Minnesota Press, Minnesota 2015)

Mayhew, E., *A Heavy Reckoning: War Medicine and Survival in Afghanistan and Beyond* (London: Profile Books, London 2017)

Novosel, M., *Dust Off: Memoirs of an Army Aviator* (Novatio, CA: Presidio, 1999)

Omori, F., *Quiet Heroes: Navy Nurses of the Korean War 1950–1953* (St Paul, MN: Smith House Press, Minnesota 2000)

Roach, P., *Citizen Surgeon: A Memoir* (Pennsauken: Book Baby, 2014)

Sharon, I., Melvan, R. and Viries, D., *Angel Walk: Nurses at War in Iraq and Afghanistan* (Brooklyn, NY: Arnica Publishing, Brooklyn 2010)

Starns, P., *Sisters of the Somme* (Stroud: The History Press, 2016)

Appendix 1

Acronyms

AECO	Aeromedical Evacuation Co-ordinating Officer
AIDS	Auto Immune Deficiency Syndrome
AIT	Air Transportable Isolator
ARDS	Acute Respiratory Distress Syndrome
ASVAT	Army Service Vocational Aptitude Test (US)
ATMIST	Age, Time of injury, Mechanism of injury, Injuries seen or suspected, Signs and Symptoms, Treatment given
BATLS	Battlefield Advanced Trauma Life Support
CASEVAC	Casualty Evacuation without Medic
CAT	Combat Application Tourniquets
CBRN	Chemical, Biological, Radiological and Nuclear
<C> ABC	Catastrophic Haemorrhage Control – Airway Breathing and Circulation
CCAST	Critical Care Air Support Team
CCATT	Critical Care Air Transport Team
CGO	Clinical Guidelines for Operations
COLPRO	Collective Protection System
CPR	Cardiopulmonary Resuscitation
CRASH	Clinical Randomisation of an Anti-fibrinolytic in Significant Haemorrhage
CSH	Combat Support Hospital
DASC	Defence Anaesthesia Simulation Course
DCR	Damage-Control Resuscitation
DCS	Damage-Control Surgery
DEPMEDS	Deployable Medical Systems
DMS	Defence Medical Services
DRIU	Damage Repair Instructional Units
DUST OFF	Dedicated Unhesitating Service to Our Fighting Forces
EAC	Early Appropriate Care
EMT	Emergency Medical Treatment
FDP	Freeze-Dried Plasma
FST	Forward Surgical Team
HEPA	High-Efficiency Particulate Air masks

HOSPEX	Hospital Exercise
ICU	Intensive Care Unit
IED	Improvised Explosive Device
LST	Landing Ship Tank
MASH	Mobile Army Surgical Hospital
MATT	Multiple Amputation Trauma Training
MEDEVAC	Medical Evacuation of Casualties
MERT	Medical Emergency Response Team
MIMMS	Major Military Incident Medical Management and Support
MOST	Military Operational Surgical Training
MPK	Micro-Processor-controlled Knee
MUST	Medical Unit Self-contained Transportable
NATO	North Atlantic Treaty Organization
NHS	National Health Service
NORMASH	Norwegian Mobile Army Surgical Hospital
NYDN	Not Yet Diagnosed Nervous
PHEC	Pre-hospital Emergency Care
PIES	Proximity, Immediacy, Expectancy and Simplicity
PTSD	Post-Traumatic Stress Disorder
RAF	Royal Air Force
RAMC	Royal Army Medical Corps
REBOA	Resuscitative Endovascular Balloon Occlusion of Aorta
RN	Royal Navy
ROTEM	Rotational Thromboelastometry
SIT	Stress Inoculation Therapy
TBI	Traumatic Brain Injury
TCCC	Tactical Combat Casualty Care
TIVA	Total Intravenous Anaesthesia
TND	Topical Negative Dressings
TRiM	Trauma Risk Management
TSAA	Tri-Service Anaesthetic Apparatus
TXA	Tranexamic Acid
UK	United Kingdom
UN	United Nations
USA	United States of America

Advances in medicine: timeline Iraq and Afghanistan

2001
- Centre of Defence Medicine established in Selly Oak to receive UK combat casualties.
- Afghanistan conflict begins. UK leads medical care in Helmand Province.

2002
- Royal status afforded to Centre of Defence Medicine.

2003
- The *Argus* from Royal Fleet Auxiliary is deployed to support tactical operations in Iraq. This ship boasted a primary casualty-receiving facility, with CT scanners, operating theatres and intensive care units.
- The formation of an Operational Emergency Department Register is introduced, which collects medical data information. The policy is introduced during the build-up of UK troops in Kuwait.
- A 25-bed field hospital accompanies troop concentrations in Iraq and is designed to follow fighting services. Bed capacity grew from 25 beds to 200 beds within 48 hours.
- UK troops in Iraq and on board the *Argus* suffer from an outbreak of gastroenteritis, severely hampering tactical operations.

2004
- Trauma Risk Management (TRiM) randomised control research trials begin.

2005
- UK military hospital at Shaibah, Iraq, installs a CT scanner.
- Eye protection introduced to prevent damage from ballistic weapons.

2006
- <C> ABC resuscitation paradigm established to replace earlier ABC paradigm.
- Combat-Application Tourniquets (CAT) introduced, along with novel haemostatic agents to stem catastrophic haemorrhage. QuikClot and Hemcon were the initial agents of choice. They have since been replaced by Celox.
- Immediate response teams are replaced by MERT.
- Digital radiology is established in field hospitals.
- First-aid drills for combat medics revised.
- Battlefield Advanced Trauma Life Support (BATLS) is revised.
- HOSPEX – a validation exercise of field hospital is held at Army Medical Service Training, York.

2007
- The first UK triple amputee, Mark Ormrod, is successfully resuscitated.
- Blood products carried on MERT aircraft.
- Clinical guidelines for operations (CGOs) are established to ensure standardised clinical care.
- Protocol for massive transfusion is established.
- Equipment introduced to enable intraosseous infusion to be performed on adults.
- Weekly Joint Theatre Clinical Case Conference is formulated.

2008
- Introduction of platelet apheresis in Afghanistan.
- More focus on mitigating hypothermia in trauma.
- UK-led tented field hospital moves to a purpose-built prefabricated medical facility in Camp Bastion.

2009
- Concept of 'right turn' resuscitation instruction is introduced, indicating that the casualty needs to go straight into operating theatre on admission.
- CGOs are updated.
- Rotational thromboelastometry (ROTEM) established to guide massive transfusion protocols.
- Weekly Pre-Hospital Emergency Care Conferences introduced.
- The Royal College of Surgeons begins Military Operational Surgical Training (MOST) courses.
- Massive transfusion protocol is reviewed.
- US supports use of Novalung to aid severely wounded UK combatant.
- Field hospital in Iraq is closed.
- RAF aeromedical team evacuate the largest cohort of wounded from Afghanistan.

2010
- Vela ventilators are introduced into field hospitals because they allow for non-invasive ventilation and offer a wide variety of ventilation options.
- To protect service personnel from perineal and genitalia injuries, often sustained as result of IED blasts, 'tier 1' pelvic ballistic protection is provided.
- Fentanyl lozenges trial begins in field hospital and forward Role-one medical facilities in Afghanistan.
- UK to Afghanistan air bridge interrupted by ash clouds.
- Renal replacement therapy (RRT) is provided for the first time in a UK field hospital.
- Royal Centre for Defence Medicine relocates to Queen Elizabeth Hospital, Birmingham.
- Help for Heroes funds a new Defence Medical Rehabilitation Unit at Headley Court.

2011
- Topical negative pressure pumps and bandages are introduced.
- Tier 2 pelvic ballistic protection provided to service personnel.
- New research facility is established by the Ministry of Defence, University Hospitals Birmingham and the University of Birmingham. The National Institute for Health Research (NIHR) Centre for Surgical Reconstruction and Microbiology aims to conduct and share medical research and innovations to advance clinical practice in battlefield medicine, and to extend this to trauma patients within the NHS.

2012
- CGOs updated.
- Belmont transfusion systems introduced in Afghanistan.
- Freeze-dried plasma (lyophilised plasma) is used in pre-hospital environment. Ministry of Defence introduces veterans' mental health programme.

2013
- Fisher House opens at the Royal Centre for Defence Medicine, to provide 'home away from home' care at the Queen Elizabeth Hospital, Birmingham.

2014
- Formal end of UK tactical combat operations in Afghanistan and Camp Bastion field hospital is closed.

Courses currently available in the UK[1]

Military Operational Surgical Training Course (MOST)

Location: Bristol

Provides individual and multidisciplinary team training, includes high-fidelity simulation, lecture-based didactic teaching, use of pro-sections and phantom limbs for regional anaesthesia training and performance of invasive skills on fresh frozen cadavers. Course is constantly updated based on evidence and current deployments.

Battlefield Advanced Trauma Life Support Course (BATLS)

Location: Defence Medical Service, Whittington, Lichfield

Focuses on modern pre-hospital care of patients in Role-one environment. Some key interventions taught include haemorrhage control with combat application tourniquets, surgical airway, needle decompressions and thoracostomy, IO access applications of pelvic and limb splints.

Medical Emergency Response Team Course (MERT)

Location: Tactical Medical Wing, RAF Brize Norton

Focuses on in-flight enhanced damage-control resuscitation. Enhanced interventions include pre-hospital RSI, blood transfusion, management of traumatic cardiac arrest and thoracotomy.

Major Military Incident Medical Management and Support Course (MIMMS)

Location: Defence Medical Services, Whittington, Lichfield

Provides a structured approach to the management of major incidents. Establishes an understanding of roles and responsibilities of multiple services responding to incidents. Promotes joint interoperability and the importance of triage.

Defence Anaesthesia Simulation Course (DASC)

Location: Centre for Simulation and Patient Safety, Health Education North West, Liverpool

Uses high-fidelity simulation training to develop an understanding of damage-control resuscitation surgery. Simulation scenarios are tailored towards contingency operations in remote environments with limited resupply and logistics. Includes use of the Tri-Service Anaesthetic Apparatus-Houghton IT. Clinical scenario debriefs are delivered with a human factor focus.

Military Advanced Paediatric Life Support Course (MAPLS)

Location: Centre for Simulation and Patient Safety, Health and Education North West, Liverpool

Uses high-fidelity simulation training to explore key challenges faced when caring for children in an operational environment. Includes familiarisation and use of the paediatric module. Difficult cases from previous operational deployments are raised to promote reflection and ethical discussions.

True Military Echo Course (TRUE)

Location: King's College London.

Use of ultrasound during damage-control surgery.

Chemical Biological, Radiation, Nuclear (CBRN) Clinical Course

Location: Defence Science and Technology Laboratory, Porton Down, Wiltshire

Damage-control resuscitation of patients exposed to chemical, biological, radiation or nuclear threats.

Index

OVERLEAF As part of the international humanitarian
response to the devastating earthquake in Haiti in 2010,
Canadian Forces initiated Operation Hestia and established
the Role 2 Enhanced No 1 Canadian Field Hospital near the
epicentre in Leogane. Supported by laboratory and x-ray
technicians, surgical teams performed 167 operations
over the course of 39 days. (Canadian Journal of Surgery,
Vol 55 No 4, August 2012)

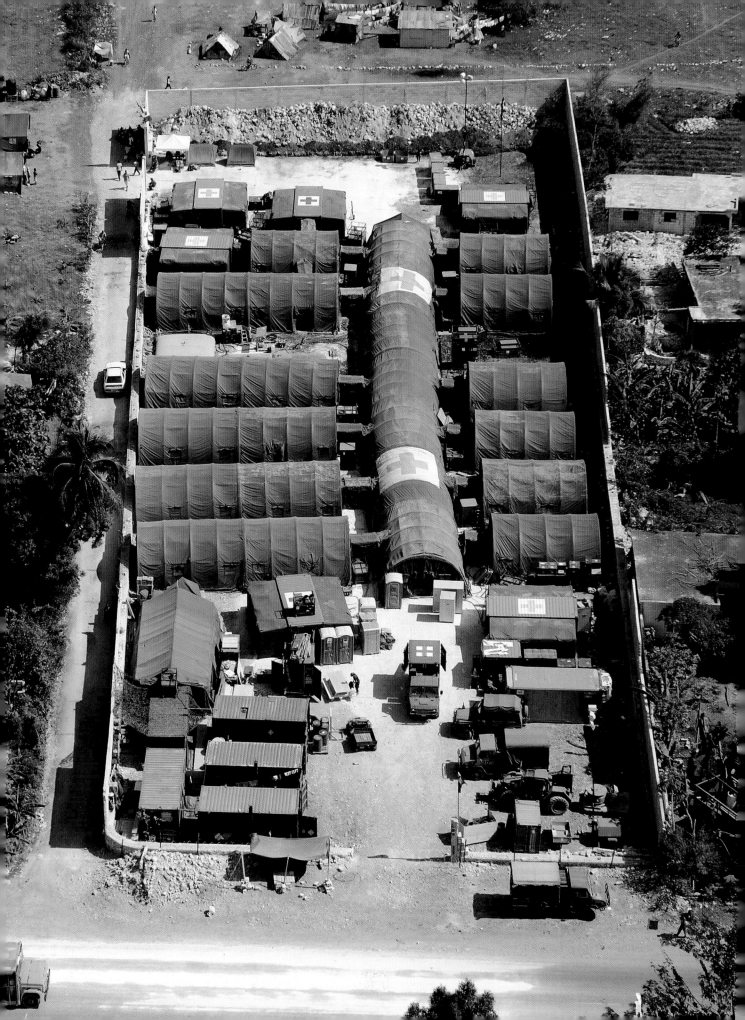